D0965483

CATHARSIS

CATHARSIS

On the Art of Medicine

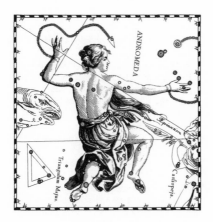

ANDRZEJ SZCZEKLIK

Translated by Antonia Lloyd-Jones
With a Foreword by Czesław Miłosz

THE UNIVERSITY OF CHICAGO PRESS
CHICAGO AND LONDON

ANDRZEJ SZCZEKLIK is professor in and chair of the Department of Medicine in the School of Medicine at the Jagiellonian University in Cracow, Poland. For his scientific contributions to the fields of asthma and myocardial infarction, he has received prestigious awards from the Royal College of Physicians, the *Lancet*, and the Foundation for Polish Science.

ANTONIA LLOYD-JONES is a freelance translator of Polish literature whose recent publications include *Mercedes-Benz*, a novel by Paweł Huelle, and *In the Garden of Memory*, a family biography by Joanna Olczak-Ronikier.

The University of Chicago Press, Chicago 60637
The University of Chicago Press, Ltd., London
© 2005 by Antonia Lloyd-Jones
All rights reserved. Published 2005
Printed in the United States of America

14 13 12 11 10 09 08 07 06 05   1 2 3 4 5

ISBN: 0-226-78869-5 (cloth)

Originally published as *Katharsis: O uzdrowicielskiej mocy natury i sztuki*
Copyright © by Andrzej Szczeklik
This translation of *Katharsis* is published by arrangement with Społeczny Instytut Wydawniczy ZNAK, Kraków (Poland).
Copyright © for the illustrations and cover design by Społeczny Instytut Wydawniczy ZNAK, 2005.

Library of Congress Cataloging-in-Publication Data

Szczeklik, Andrzej.
    [Katharsis. English]
    Catharsis : on the art of medicine / Andrzej Szczeklik ; translated by Antonia Lloyd-Jones ; with a foreword by Czeslaw Milosz.
        p. cm.
    Includes bibliographical references.
    ISBN 0-226-78869-5 (cloth : alk. paper)
    1. Medicine—Philosophy. 2. Medicine—History. 3. Catharsis.
    4. Medicine—Miscellanea. I. Title.

R723.S9413 2005
610′.1—dc22

                                                                 2005043732

♾ The paper used in this publication meets the minimum requirements of the American National Standard for Information Sciences— Permanence of Paper for Printed Library Materials, ANSI Z39.48-1992.

CONTENTS

Czesław Miłosz

There are two sides involved: the patient's and the doctor's. We all fall ill at various stages of life, and the experience of being a patient is universal. But when we are ill, who is the person who comes so close to us, and whose words carry so much weight? We hang on his lips as he utters statements that may be of life-or-death importance. Admittedly, we invest him with a power that he might not actually possess. To us he is a magus, a shaman, or at any rate someone whose profession raises him above us ordinary mortals.

Dr. Szczeklik's book tells us about the art of medicine. He admits that it is a skill derived from magic and that it is actually hard to define, because elements of both art and science are inseparably combined within it. From this book we learn about the endless doubts and questions that arise in the mind of the powerful magus, and about his frequent lack of confidence in his own strengths. At the same time, however, Dr. Szczeklik writes about the incredible rarity of a truly Great Doctor, whose colleagues regard him with reverential awe because unlike them he only has to look at a patient to know what is wrong.

In fact, this book also shows us medicine from the historical perspective and its surprisingly late focus on the wonders of the human organism. William Harvey discovered the circulation of the blood in the early seventeenth century, while we owe our awareness of the existence of such a thing as bacteria to Louis Pasteur, who in the second half of the nineteenth century made an accidental discovery that was the start of modern immunology.

One of the book's merits is its copious reference to the literature of centuries past. Dr. Szczeklik quotes Petrarch, for example, who claimed six hundred years ago that if you were to take a thousand people suffering from a given illness, hand half of them over to the mercy of doctors, and leave the other half to themselves, the ones left on their own would have a greater chance of recovery. Relatively recently, in a statement by Harvard biochemist Lawrence J. Henderson dating from 1910, a sick person who went to see a doctor had a not much more than 50% chance of recovery — slightly better than in Petrarch's day, but not much.

Dr. Szczeklik is conscious of writing about his own profession rather in the way that a shaman would, that is, without revealing all the secrets known only to a small number of ideal doctors, as the skill of making a correct diagnosis eludes purely rational expression. There is also a mysterious connection between the human organism and some spiritual energies, thanks to which science alone cannot answer many of our questions about ourselves. So perhaps the author is right to use the word *katharsis,* or "purification," and to go back to ancient Greek drama, in which the chorus, combining music and dance, poetry and song, served to purify the soul. This way of referring back to the ancient world makes us think about the age-old continuity of the medical profession, which quite possibly derives its high standing from its permanent place on the border between life and death.

I should add that Dr. Szczeklik does not limit himself to terribly serious comments, although his humor is dry and restrained. For example, when he is describing the fundamental professional duty of saving life, he says: "When I was just starting out as a doctor, and Wrocław was in the grip of the worst winter of the century, at three in the morning a frozen man was brought in to us at the hospital. He had been found by the river Oder, where the temperature was down to minus 35°C. He was as stiff and cold as an icicle, he wasn't breathing, and his heart had stopped. The electrocardiogram showed a straight, horizontal line. The idea of reanimation had only just entered the debate, and we had no equipment at all. There were only two of us, myself and a nurse. I began to massage the heart, while she tried mouth-to-mouth resuscitation. With each breath the room was filled with the fumes of methylated spirits. The man's heart started functioning again after about an hour's massage, and the breathing shortly after. The next day the patient walked out on his own two feet, having earlier upbraided us for losing his packet of extra-strength cigarettes."

In the practice of an experienced doctor an incident like that one is unusual, yet it is the sort of encounter that prompts us to dress our doctor in the full regalia of a magus, even if the patient who is brought back to life can only remember that he had a packet of extra-strengths.

Andrzej Szczeklik is a doctor with profound knowledge of the humanities, in whom poets and artists sense a kindred mentality, though it relies on erudition unfamiliar to them, from the fields of microbiology, chemistry, and genetics. Nowadays, as we debate the crucial issue of moral limits, imposed on us by the progress of science, a book by a doctor who is also educated in the humanities and is sensitive to the problems involved is highly desirable and interesting.

CATHARSIS

I. RIBBONS

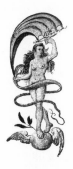

This is the net, as old as this world, eternal.
It falls from heaven to earth in circles.
It surrounds and envelops everything in existence.
It joins us in its embrace and enfolds us in necessity.

Necessity bears the name Ananke. We are all subject to her, even the gods on Olympus. She is the only one whom Homer did not personify in human form, which is why we doubt if she had a face. He presented only her daughter, Fate, who spins the thread of life. In Hesiod's version there are three Fates: the first one works the spindle, the second keeps an eye on the length of the thread, and the third sits waiting with the shears in her hands. Above them, shrouded in the utmost mystery, towers Ananke, from whose verdict there is no recall, and whom Aeschylus called "the strong Fate."

In ancient Greece many people used to question the existence of the gods, but no one ever doubted the existence of the net, whose might was greater than that of the gods. After all, it was invisible. The twinkling trail of it could be seen in the sky as the Milky Way and was also faithfully reproduced in miniature in the girdle slung across the hips of Aphrodite, "in which all charms and spells reside," cast upon mankind. And so the Milky Way, that girdle of the night, cast like a bright streak across the darkness of the sky, changed into a deception on the body of Aphrodite. As if "a soft, deceiving sash should cover the inflexible bond of necessity."

We have the "eyewitness account" of a traveler on the astral highways who reached the very beginning of the net. The story is told by Er, the hero of one of Plato's finest legends, appearing at the end of his *Republic*. It took him twelve days to reach a place from where the Spindle of Necessity was visible. There before his eyes appeared "a shaft of light, like a pillar, extending from above through the whole heaven and earth. The light was more like a rainbow than anything else, only brighter and more pure." The spindle was driven by eight cosmic circles, on each of which lived a Siren. The eight Sirens sang to the rhythm of the revolutions of the cosmic whorl "to produce one single harmony." This was the very spot where the Fates, the parthenogenetic daughters of Necessity, were busily at work. Here at their hearth the souls of the dead, wandering in the afterworld, drew their lots, determining their next incarnation after the time of Judgment. Everything was suffused with the brightness that marked the beginning of the shining net.

The net connects heaven and earth and unites earthly beings with one another. This joining of everything to everything else remains hidden from our sight. If people had to see the net the whole time, they would be unable to bear the sight of it. They would immediately become tangled in it and would suffocate. Only in rare moments of respite does the memory of it return. It happens when something destroys our neutral attitude, when we extricate ourselves from worldly monotony, when the intensity of life increases "through honor or death, victory or sacrifice, marriage or prayer, initiation or possession, purification or mourning, anything and everything that stirred a person and demanded a meaning." This sort of an experience may be lying in wait for us at any place and at any time. A story from Ireland offers a marvelous example. According to the legend, one day Saint Kevin was kneeling down to pray with his arms outstretched in the form of a cross at Glendalough in the Wicklow Mountains. A blackbird mistook his hand for a branch, landed, laid eggs in it, and started to nest. Rather than disturb the bird, Kevin stayed immobile, holding out his hands, until the eggs hatched and the fledglings grew wings—"true to life, if subversive to common sense." For weeks he prayed on his knees, "a prayer his body makes entirely . . . , finding himself linked into the network of eternal life."

Shortly before any religious festival, on Polish roads and lanes colored ribbons start fluttering in the wind. It is children who tie them to the branches of trees and bushes, and to the tops of wayside chapels. Similarly, thousands of years ago, to grace their infrequent festive occasions the Greeks used to tie ribbons around the torsos of victorious Olympic athletes, on the bows of ships and the arms of statues. What were those ribbons fluttering in the wind, those "vain, winged tassels"? A brief appearance in our world by the net, a reminder of our common fate, of the bonds that link everything with everything else, a revelation of the thread of the fabric that gives our life a meaning.

We live in a universe whose deepest layers are formed by the quantum system. Quantum structures shape reality at the atomic and the subatomic levels; they do it in a way that is outside our daily experience and goes against our intuitions born of common sense. Thus, the components of the quantum system are mysteriously "entangled," so that some are aware of others. The word "entangled" is not a rhetorical figure of speech, but a technical term in physics. The entanglement of the quantum system means that it is a perfect whole, and that the very subtlest manipulation of any of its parts immediately has an effect on the rest of it. "And that happens regardless of spatial distance: two photons can create an entangled system even when they are at opposite ends of a supercluster of galaxies" — just as if the quantum world were entwined in an eternal net, the one that surrounds, envelops, and enfolds us in necessity.

Etymology tells us that the name Ananke contains echoes of "constriction" and also "kinship." The same sort of double semantic meaning is rendered by the word "bonds." An alternative view finds a close relation between the word *ananke* and the phrase "taking in one's arms." This duality, or antagonism even, finds its reflection in the net of Necessity. Inevitably, inexorably it tightens around mankind, as the world atomizes and scurries aside. But the pressure of the net falls as it comes closer, as we discover the bonds linking us with others, and the thread becomes a thread of mutual understanding, sympathy, and trust. This can happen unexpectedly, and then it is like a spark jumping between two electrodes, like the flash of a metaphor joining distant words together. In that flash an affinity is revealed, and the net starts shining with all the stars in the Milky Way. Medicine is the process of discovering that affinity.

In every profession there are fundamental situations that reveal its inner core. In medicine it is an encounter between two people, the patient and the doctor. The patient might, for example, be a woman from the highlands who spent her first night in a hospital only after passing the age of seventy. How many things must she find amazing, or funny, how much must frighten her, like the illness she came in with. Another time the patient is someone seen in a hurry at a clinic, who is burdened with numerous discouraging experiences of contact with medicine. The people change and the scenery changes, from Accident and Emergency to the Out-patient Department, from the consulting room to the hospital ward, but the situation remains the same—it is an encounter between two people: patient and doctor.

Along comes the patient with his pain, affliction, suffering, or anxiety and asks for help. His request is rarely literal, of course—it has various forms of expression. It might be a stream of words, to stave off the anxiety, or stony facial features that conceal a lack of trust in the doctor. So the patient tells his story, while the doctor has to listen, to hear his tale. Now and then he has to ask a question to avoid losing the plot, uncover a relevant detail, or get a precise chronology. For the person doing the telling, this case history is of the utmost importance. The person doing the listening should also remember that one day one of these stories will be his own, one of these illnesses will affect the doctor too. But will he recognize it when it happens? A young medic, with no experience, is always suspecting that he has got one of the countless diseases he has heard about. What about an experienced doctor? He has a better chance of making a correct self-diagnosis, as long as his experience, that "beacon on the seashore, that a man aims for on a cloudy day," has not turned into "cotton in the ears to stop the sound of human groaning."

The first conversation with the patient, the medical interview to gather information about the illness, is known to doctors as "taking the history," which in Europe we often call the anamnesis. This name is a reference to Plato, and although the exact nuance of Plato's anamnesis was slightly different, and its sense deeper, it was in fact the most vital and original means of gaining knowledge. Similarly in the art of medicine it is of crucial significance to gaining knowledge of an illness.

In Plato the anamnesis was the first source of knowledge, coming ahead of perception. Isn't it the same in medicine? Before the doctor starts to "perceive" what is wrong, before he proceeds with his examination, his tapping and listening, and all other such activities that we call "the objective examination," he listens to a story from the past. With a skillful word here and there he helps to bring to light some knowledge that is a piece of history, a recollection. He also needs to be curious about the case history, so that the patient feels that someone, maybe for the very first time, is truly interested in his misfortune. The doctor has to talk the same language as the patient. Sometimes the rhythm of speech and the tone of voice can steer him toward the right diagnosis. A rapid salvo of sentences, racing each other, as if urged on by damp, fidgeting hands, an anxious or even disturbed tone make him think of an overactive thyroid. A hoarse, low voice, emerging slowly from a swollen face with a waxy tinge tells him that the same gland is underactive. All he has to do is listen. And only occasionally is the help of a third person necessary . . .

Before the war my father, a doctor, was summoned to the suburban estate of Prince X, who had been taken ill. The prince was sitting in a tall armchair, with his valet Jan standing right behind him. While the doctor is gathering information, toward the end of a litany of questions that he asks, there is usually a final one about past illnesses of the sort that might perhaps be termed embarrassing. My father asked this question. There was a resounding silence, until finally the prince leaned back a little and asked: "Jan, that time in Paris, was that it?" "No, nothing like that, your Highness," came the reply. "No, nothing like that, Doctor," replied the prince.

And so the doctor enters the patient's world, which often includes content that is intimate, forgotten or hidden from his immediate circle, or even from himself. In some cases, such as schizophrenia, this world may be full of mysterious energies, both good and bad forces, or may have been pervaded by wavelengths that control human behavior. "Beneath the ordinary picture of the world a different one lies hidden," wrote the distinguished Polish psychiatrist Antoni Kępiński in his work on schizophrenia. The patient is convinced he has discovered the true essence of reality, while the rest of us are aware of only its surface appearance. How hard it is to break through to this world and to access it—unless you are very lucky.

When I took my psychiatry exam, the professor led me into a spacious room. "Please report to me once you have got the anamnesis," he said and left the room, closing the door, which had no handle on the inside. There by a barred window, wearing striped hospital pyjamas, a man was standing straight, still as a statue, on one leg. He was holding the other one up, bent at the knee and not moving. His eyes were extremely wide open and he was staring into space, as if frozen solid at some point in time. Nothing I did made him react, although I tried saying things, offering him a cigarette, talking about the latest football results, humming and whistling tunes, and imitating a cat meowing and a dog barking. He was unmoved by my pleas that my exam result depended on a few words from him. "Too bad," I thought. "Old Kant was right, we're surrounded by *Ding an sich*, unrecognizable phenomena, things that exist purely in themselves." So I turned my back on my stylite friend and began mechanically serving balls on a Ping-Pong table set up in another corner of the room. One, two, one, two, went the celluloid balls, tapping out a steady rhythm as they jumped from my field of play into my absent opponent's. Suddenly—was that a thump? I turned around. The raised leg had come back to earth. "Shall we play?" I heard. He was an excellent player. In the third set he suggested we switch to a first-name basis. What amazing things he then told me! I had no trouble passing the exam.

The rhythmical tap of a Ping-Pong ball had broken the silence in which the patient was locked. Something had been opened. Searching for the keys that would open the gates of anamnesis occupied the minds of the ancient Greeks, because anamnesis was the only way to reach the superior state of being that Plato discovered, the world of Ideas. Thus, Greek thought went back to archaic myth, to the time before birth, to what Mircea Eliade defines as the *illud tempus,* when "the soul was directly contemplating Ideas. . . . Man had to remember this time if he was to know the *truth* and participate in Being."

In medicine the recollection does not have to reach so far back, only to the beginning of the illness, though it tries to investigate the very first symptoms, hovers about in the border zone, and crosses into another, earlier world, the world of good health, the world without illness. This process is encumbered nowadays, since many barriers have been broken and the sphere of interhuman relations is free of any standard principles. One's position with regard to the other person has changed. "We simply don't know what can be expected of the Other." Thus, it is harder to reveal oneself, as there are too many dangerous unknowns in the air. And yet without this process medicine cannot exist. Of course, the basic conditions have to be met: the doctor cannot judge the patient or censure him, but can try to understand him and help him. He should be open to anyone who has succumbed to the particular pressure of solitude. In difficult situations the doctor turns to the most secret arcana of his art, in order to connect the thread of understanding and discover the bonds that link two people. May his reward—at special moments—be the flutter of ribbons in the wind.

II. CONSTELLATIONS

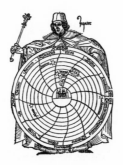

Medicine and art are descended from the same roots. They both originated in magic—a practice based on the omnipotence of the word. A correctly uttered magic spell can bring health or death, rain or drought, call up the spirits or reveal the future. It can activate connections that are invisible to those who are calmly and confidently absorbed in everyday affairs. Incantations used to "break spells and ward off illness . . . are in the form of verse, full of alliteration and assonance, in every respect worth the attention of those who study literature."

The art of the word, assisted by experience accumulated by generations of priests and doctors, enabled mankind to recover its place in the cosmos, which right up to the seventeenth and eighteenth centuries echoed with harmony. The sense of an analogy between the structure and rhythm of the cosmos and the rhythms of mankind, between the macrocosmos and the microcosmos, as they would later be named, inspired philosophers and doctors for over two millennia. Man was in concord with the cosmos. Illness was a disturbance of this concord, a break with harmony, a dissonance.

This notion has come back again and again as a myth in numerous versions. To Hippocrates illness appeared to be "a disorder that disfigures beauty, and which it is the physician's task to remove." Hippocrates too called medicine an art, *techne*. In the sixteenth century Paracelsus saw a spiritual connection within the cosmos joining all things with one another. He taught that the universe was a living thing that undergoes the same phases of development as organisms on earth. Anticipating knowledge about the astral origin of our body parts, he wrote that man is a microcosmos built of the very same elements as the macrocosmos, that is, the universe. He saw the divine life element within us as the "archeus" or "inner alchemist" (*innewendige Alchemist*). It controlled the body and separated the positive things in our food from the harmful ones. Illness was caused by alien spiritual forces taking over the archeus. Through medical treatment it could be liberated from constraint—thanks to nature, to whose succor came an art that had mysteries at its command.

If we should happen to smile with gentle indulgence at these attempts to grasp the essence of illness, let us not forget that to this day we still find it a difficult business. In 1972 a group of world experts on asthma held a meeting at a beautiful mountain resort. They were given one single task: to give the illness a definition. A week later they parted ways without having achieved their goal. Since that time the leading international bodies have twice already issued diametrically different definitions of asthma. Yet in practice a doctor generally has no trouble at all in diagnosing it. He quite often does so before putting his stethoscope to the patient's lungs—he only has to hear his protracted, wheezing exhalation. Its echo resounds in the onomatopoeic word "asthma." Homer used it for the first time in his description of the fallen Hector, lying prostrate under the walls of Troy in terrible breathlessness (*asthmati*). Doesn't the prefix "Ha! (-sthma)" sound like the protracted breath of an asthmatic?

To diagnose an illness we rely on the symptoms, not on its

causes and the way it arose, which are so difficult to define. In the simplest situation we seek out the dominant symptom and associate it with one of the more common illnesses. As the British saying goes, "If you hear the sound of hooves, look round for a horse, because zebras are very rare." But sometimes the situation is more complicated. The changeability, instability, similarity and fleeting nature of symptoms can make reaching a diagnosis rather like Hamlet's conversation with Polonius as they watch the clouds:

HAMLET: Do you see yonder cloud that's almost in shape of a camel.
POLONIUS: By th' mass and 'tis, like a camel indeed.
HAMLET: Methinks it is like a weasel.
POLONIUS: It is back'd like a weasel.
HAMLET: Or like a whale.
POLONIUS: Very like a whale.

The encounter with the patient, their conversation, the anamnesis and examination immerse the doctor in a world of signals sent by the sick person's organism. The doctor has to develop within himself a particular kind of sensitivity so that these signals will not pass him by, but get through to him. When they do, in a single instant they can combine to form a constellation of symptoms that he can interpret to make his diagnosis of the illness.

This constellation of symptoms is like a constellation of stars in the sky, showing a sailor the way into port. It defines his position on the map, dispels the darkness, and lulls his sense of insecurity. Just as in a dream, when all of a sudden the strange, unfamiliar person we've been dreaming about half the night turns out to be someone we know well. That instant, that flash of change from the unknown into the familiar—that's what diagnosis is.

Sophocles describes the scene where Orestes encounters his sister, Electra, over the urn that supposedly contains his ashes. At first he takes her for a slave girl, but later on he recognizes her by her tears. He tells her the urn is empty and reveals his true identity. They are both overcome with joy. This theme runs through the dreams and myths of many nations: we think the person standing before us is a stranger, but actually he is the person we love the most.

The finest incident of this kind happened when two of the apostles were on their way to Emmaus, a village near Jerusalem. Jesus came up, walked along with them, and talked to them. "But their eyes were held from recognizing Him." Only at the inn, "when He had reclined at table with them, He happened to take bread and utter a blessing; He broke it and offered it to them. Then their eyes were opened, and they recognized Him; but He vanished from their sight. And they admitted to each other: 'Were not our hearts on fire within us, as He was speaking to us on the road and opened to us the sense of the Scriptures!'"

In Velázquez's painting, the first person to recognize Him at the inn, before the apostles do, is the black servant girl. She is in the kitchen, carrying a jar of wine to bring to the table where they have sat down to their bread, when the certainty comes over her. Was it not He

> who had looked at her, once, across the crowd,
> as no one ever had looked?
> Had seen her? Had spoken as if to her?

The doctor's road to Emmaus sometimes seems endless. When eighteen-year-old Basia N. was brought to us from a remote village in the Opole region, at first sight her case looked pedestrian. Six months earlier she had injured her leg, which had been suppurating ever since. She had already been in several hospitals, where no one had succeeded in controlling the infection. Was it a case of exceptionally virulent bacteria? Or some sort of disorder in a young organism's immune system? We could find nothing to confirm either of these theories. Meanwhile the patient had a daily temperature of up to 40°C, her leg was covered in more and more new abscesses, kept swelling up, and was approaching monstrous dimensions, but we were getting nowhere. Our helplessness was weighing on us more and more, so we began to seek advice. After a detailed examination a brilliant local surgeon and a superb pathologist diagnosed the sick leg as having a congenital disorder affecting the development of the blood vessels. Their evidence did not fully convince us, but we had nothing better to suggest. Over the course of a year we sent our patient to be treated at eight reputable hospitals within Poland. Sometimes she came back with an improvement, but after a couple of weeks her fever would flare up, and the initial, tiny abscesses would appear on her leg. We were afraid of a heart attack or sepsis. We had no idea how to help this extremely unwell, quiet and introverted, pretty girl. Once I found her reading a book called *How to Become a Giant* and managed to draw her into conversation. I found out about the attractive studies and beautiful home awaiting her, which her rich brother was supposed to be taking care of, though he never came to visit her in hospital.

In desperation, I referred the case to a friend who is a professor of cardiology in London. He made the decision to take her on, though he had no new theory to propose. We approached the Ministry of Health for permission to have the patient treated abroad. Meanwhile, fearing the worst, we transferred her to a surgical hospital in Katowice. I asked the professor there to keep a particularly close eye on her. Ten days later he called and said: "Just like our predecessors we have made a deep incision the entire length of the leg and extracted a bucketful of pus. Can we send her back to you in a week's time? As for the cause, I'd consider Münchhausen's." Münchhausen's? We had thought about it a year ago, and at the time we had doubled our observation, but we hadn't found any evidence. Soon after she came back from Katowice her symptoms sharply intensified, and the duty surgeon summoned in the night rather unexpectedly wrapped the entire leg in plaster. When I examined it two days later, the plaster had made touching the leg impossible, but for the first time a blister had appeared on her hand, clearly heralding the development of an abscess. At the center of the blister I could see the tiny mark of a pinprick. So it was Münchhausen's!

Karl Friedrich Hieronymus Baron von Münchhausen (1720–1797) was a German officer in the pay of the Russians who fought against the Turks before settling in Hannover, where over a glass of wine he enjoyed entertaining his friends with the story of his adventures. Their boundless improbability and absurdity, interspersed with apt, highly probable facts, gained him incredible popularity. "The Lying Baron" (*Der Lügenbaron*), as he was known, would tell you how he had dragged himself out of a quagmire by pulling as hard as he could on his own hair, or about the time he hit a deer between the horns with a cherry stone, only to run into it again years later with a cherry tree growing from its forehead.

In 1951 a British doctor suggested the name "Münchhausen's syndrome" for patients displaying an incredible wealth of bizarre and dramatic symptoms that do not easily fit together into a meaningful set, but form unusual constellations. These patients drift from hospital to hospital, willingly submitting to the most elaborate diagnostic and therapeutic procedures, including frequent major operations. The entire illness is the result of repeated self-mutilation, performed so cunningly and secretly, and causing such immense suffering, that it leads experienced doctors up the garden path. It is a psychological illness that imposes compulsive behavior on the patient, most definitely outside his sphere of consciousness. Discovering the reason for his illness and revealing the truth to the patient causes him to disappear for ever from the field of perception of the doctor who has done so. Our quiet, enigmatic Basia was prepared to set off on more hospital journeys but sank into silent rage at the thought that she might end up at the Katowice hospital where she had been told that maybe she was injecting the infection into her own leg. So the gifted psychiatrist with whom I started treating her jointly adopted a strategy whereby in no circumstances would we ever mention blame or fraud, but instead we would acknowledge the patient as the bearer of a mystery that we were trying to fathom, by referring to her mother, family, and close friends. Will it be effective? Shall we succeed? The statistics do not inspire optimism, but we are consoled by the fact that there are no two similar patients with Münchhausen's syndrome. But how can you really get through to someone who has chosen suffering as the ultimate solution to life's problems?

Münchhausen's syndrome is extremely unusual. However, it is not quite so uncommon for a doctor to feel increasingly helpless as he grapples with a particular illness, at a time when the treatment isn't working. The pile of clinical notes grows higher, and ever more detailed and elaborate examinations are made, but there is no progress whatsoever. Driven close to extreme measures, we call in someone very special. We can imagine the scene: a hospital room where there's a patient with some fundamental problems. The ward round begins, and the specially invited doctor comes in, followed by a long queue of people in white coats. The most senior of them gives the visitor a report on the history of the illness and all their findings so far. Meanwhile he stands there and listens. Someone is probably thinking: "Is he really listening?" Then he takes a look at the patient, touches him, puts his stethoscope to his chest, and finally says: "This is a case of so and so. You have to do such and such." And he proves correct. Suddenly everything changes. As in *katharsis*, a process of purification follows, and that's when the doctor in charge of the patient, who has gone through weeks on end, sometimes months of anguish, trying to find a solution but getting nowhere, thinks about that unusual guest and says: "What a Great Doctor!"

This scene contains something magical that has its roots in the mists of medical prehistory. The Great Doctor is almost as much a rarity as Münchhausen's syndrome. You encounter only two or three at most in a long professional career. They remind you of people blessed with perfect pitch, who hear notes the way the rest of us see colors. Just as you recognize the color yellow without a second thought, and do not mistake it for red, they can immediately distinguish the sound of F from G. A Great Doctor moves about in the world of illness just as freely as a person with perfect pitch does within tonal space, which is inaccessible to others.

The doctor is at a loss whenever he is unable to name an illness, cannot understand the "confession of the body," cannot grasp why something is happening in a particular way, or doesn't know how to help. His helplessness soon stops being purely his private concern. After all, it affects the patient and his immediate circle. Luckily, there are also cases where the diagnosis is handed to you on a plate, including the course of action to take. It was a beautiful day in spring when we finally opened the intensive care unit. Despite all sorts of problems we had managed to do it—the first such unit in Cracow! There we stood, three doctors, on the first floor, outside our as yet empty unit, bursting with youth and strength. We felt as if nothing on earth was impossible, and we were full of anticipation, extremely excited about the coming events that would allow us to show off our unusual skills.

Then a man appeared on the ground floor and began to clamber up the stairs toward us; in that old ruin of a hospital none of the elevators were working. He was entirely dressed in black, and one of us said: "He's well prepared for this occasion!" He was on his way back from his mother-in-law's funeral, where he had felt unwell and decided to look in at the nearest hospital. Out of breath, he dragged himself up the stairs and fell at our feet—dead. Just what we'd been waiting for—what luck! We threw ourselves upon him.

Two weeks later when our first patient was on his way home,

the nurses gave him some flowers, and bidding us farewell he said: "Wherever she is, my mother-in-law'll drop dead all over again when she sees how lightly I got off!"

"Coming events cast their shadows before," in the words of Jacobite poet Thomas Campbell's famous warning. On that bright spring day, as we stood outside the newly opened intensive care unit, so full of expectations, did we notice the shadow lying before the man in black as he was coming toward us? Or even earlier, as he was making his way from the cemetery to the hospital? No, all we felt was blissfully ignorant hope for the coming of events. We did not have the sort of knowledge of the future that could have revealed a correct clinical diagnosis. How far can we be sure about such knowledge? How much of this do we have the right and the duty to tell the patient? In this respect, for centuries physicians consulted the Sibyls, or oracles.

To this day in Delphi you can see the rock above a precipice where Phemonoe, daughter of Apollo, foretold the future as the first Sibyl, known as the Pythia. Dressed in a simple tunic, she sat on a tripod and greeted those who entered the temple with her gaze. Vapors came pouring from a crevice in the ground, and the so-called umbilical stone, wrapped in the cords of a double net, marked the center of the world. Here too grew a laurel tree "whose leaves think" and which if chewed increased the oracle's prophetic gift. Beside her stood a golden statue of Apollo; behind her a stream of water trickled by and a snake kept watch—the source of the Pythia's strength.

The Pythia's predictions were enigmatic, abstruse even. When Croesus consulted the Delphic oracle from his faraway kingdom before taking the momentous step of declaring war on Cyrus, king of Persia, she gave him a truly ambiguous reply: "You will destroy a great empire." Croesus assumed she meant Cyrus's empire, but actually it was his kingdom that she had in mind. Old and defeated, taken prisoner by Cyrus, Croesus sent a final gift to Delphi: his chains. There was only one man who consulted the oracle and got no reply—when Alexander the Great stood before the Pythia she was silent.

For many long centuries all those who visited the oracle to divine the secrets of their lives heard words whose meaning they understood only after the event. The Sibyls—the women inspired by the god—spoke in perfect verse. The hexameter was Apollo's gift to his daughter Phemonoe. "Poetry thus arrived on the scene as the form structuring . . . ambiguous words." Is that why poetry is so equivocal by nature? And is that why "the language of the immortals must differ from the language of men"? Is it for the same simple reason that mankind cannot bear an out-and-out mystery? So too perhaps the patient doesn't want—and ought not—to hear the whole, cruel truth from the doctor all at once.

> Tell all the truth but tell it slant—
> Success in Circuit lies
> Too bright for our infirm Delight
> The Truth's superb surprise
> As Lightning to the Children eased
> With explanation kind
> The Truth must dazzle gradually
> Or every man be blind—

On his native island of Kos, only about three hundred kilometers from Delphi, Hippocrates did not consult the oracle to seek out the harbingers of fate, but looked at his patient's features instead. He knew what to seize upon. He wrote that in our short life "making pronouncements is difficult," because "the opportunities are short-lived" and "experience can be deceptive." Yet he was able, as no one before him, to see the shadow of death on a patient's face when it was standing by and high in the sky the shears were already closing on the thread. Ever since, every generation of doctors has looked through his eyes, recognizing the *facies hippo-cratica* just as he represented it: "a pointed nose, sunken eyes, concave temples, cold ears that are shrunken and everted, the skin around the brow hard, taut, and dry, the color of the whole face a pallid green, black, livid, or leaden."

Hippocrates took his prognosis to a masterly level in his famous aphorisms. For example, he wrote: "A spasm occurring on top of a wound is fatal," quite certainly with tetanus in mind. And again: "In cases of jaundice it is a bad symptom when the liver becomes hardened," most probably thinking of liver cancer. Or finally: "Any swelling that appears after a severe illness is bad," referring to an inflammation of the kidneys or heart failure. A doctor who makes an accurate prediction or unerringly presents a prognosis or final outcome instantly gains admiration and acclaim. A correct prognosis has always made a great impression, even on other doctors. It was once seen as a mysterious talent, evidence of excellence in one's art. When Wojciech Baza, court doctor to King Zygmunt the Old, went to visit Paracelsus in Basel, he was dazzled by the incredible self-confidence with which the illustrious Swiss physician predicted a recovery. He was called to a patient whom some other doctors had already pronounced dead. Paracelsus examined the dying man and invited him to dine with him the next day. Sure enough, shortly after, the patient got up from his bed and came to dinner. For all his astounding magic, Paracelsus was the descendant of Hippocrates, someone who had read his aphorisms or added nuances to them himself.

Illustriously famous as a magician, this miracle-working doctor, the prototype for Faust, cured eighteen kings and princes when all other doctors had abandoned them. Though he defended his doctorate at Ferrara, he sought the company of barbers, shepherds, blacksmiths, Gypsies, and old women, from whom he learned the occult art of healing. He even went to see the universally despised executioner, who set limbs. A restless spirit, Paracelsus traveled about on horseback and spent his nights writing. By his side he wore a sword with an opening pommel hollowed out of the hilt, where he kept pills for the sick. There was also a rumor that he carried a devil in there. He practiced his art in more and more different countries and knew the secret powers in every one of them. Among them he placed the highest value on the power of the stars, and said: "He who does not take control of the stars, shall be ruled by the stars at their own will." These words echo with the belief that the stars over the horizon at the time of a man's birth will shape his fate. "If you follow your star, you will inevitably sail to a splendid port."

According to science, our fate is not written in the stars, but in our genes. In a few exceptional cases only it is one single gene, but usually others are linked with it in proximity, and so are some far-off genes, on distant chromosomes. When stimulated they will come together to shine with a single light; they can herald asthma or, in a different configuration, some other illness. The decisive factor is the set they form, their configuration or constellation, just as a constellation of stars over the horizon was supposed to herald the fate of a new arrival in the world.

So nowadays it is inside ourselves, in our genes, rather than in the sky, that we look for prerecorded information about our future. As our genetic constellations are of celestial provenance, maybe gaining knowledge of them will recreate a lost bond with the sky, show us the way back, and restore a vanished harmony.

III. THE ELIXIR
OF LIFE

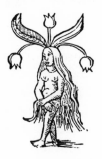

The birth of medicine is marked by love and fire. Apollo's love for Coronis—a violent, overwhelming love. When Coronis was pregnant with Apollo's child, she was unfaithful to him with a foreigner. Apollo's envoy, a white crow, was keeping watch on her. At once it flew to its master and, as spies are in the habit of doing, denounced his lover's infidelity to him. In his anger Apollo threw his plectrum at the crow, and glared at it with such hatred that its feathers turned black as pitch forever after. Then he appealed to his sister Artemis to kill his faithless lover with an arrow from her bow. As she was dying, Coronis just managed to whisper to the god that by killing her he was also killing his own son. When her body was laid out on a funeral pyre as high as a city wall, and the flames were starting to engulf it, Apollo tore the child from her womb by Caesarean section. And so Asclepius came into the world, "the health-giver," also known as the patron or god of medicine. He spent many long years as the pupil of the good centaur Chiron, who first sowed healing herbs in Thessaly. Thanks to him, Asclepius gained such great skill as a healer that many years later he was bold enough to restore the dead to life, for which Zeus struck him with a thunderbolt. Thus, the first god of medicine was reduced to ashes—a deity who had arisen from the ashes, all that was left of his mother's body on the burning pyre at the moment when he came into the world. By resurrecting the dead and restoring life Asclepius had overstepped the bounds of the human span of existence, and for this transgression he was consumed by fire.

Yet mankind did not renounce the dreams personified by Asclepius. From the dawn of time people have sought ways of healing their wounds, driving away illness, and restoring health. They turned to plants in an attempt to extract their secret powers. They used willow bark to ease fever and aching joints, resin for painful cramps and anxiety, and thyme for coughs and infections. They also studied animals and followed the example of the dog that licks its wounds by bathing their own in water. In Egypt they came upon the idea of applying enemas when they saw how the ibis, after a copious meal, would turn its head, using its long neck and curved beak to rinse its alimentary canal with water from behind. We also owe the words "pharmacy" and "pharmacology" to the Egyptians, as they are derived from *ph-ar-maki,* meaning "that which protects." Plants had secret powers; both health and death lay hidden in them. If a substance could heal, in a higher dose it could kill. Sometimes the most potent healing properties were concealed in only one part of a plant, such as the mandragora root, which gave a piercing shriek as it was pulled from the ground. Sometimes there were a large number of substances in a medicine. Theriac, which enjoyed unflagging popularity for two millennia, included eighty-nine ingredients, from opium to animal products including powdered snake. But above all, for thousands of years mankind sought the Philosopher's Stone, the *quinta essentia,* the *elixir vitae.* It was being sought in China many centuries before Christ, and the search continued all the way to

Newton and beyond. The Philosopher's Stone, identified with the elixir of life, was supposed to cleanse the body of all illness, turn base metal into gold ore, prolong life by hundreds of years, and restore youth to the elderly. This myth of a miraculous plant, a potion of immortality, the secret of life held enchanted in a stone was the dream of all the Indo-European peoples.

No one dreamed this dream more ardently than the alchemists. Although many of the trends in alchemy were derived from Greek philosophy, with Egyptian, Persian, and Chinese elements added in Hellenistic Alexandria, it reached its apogee at the turn of the sixteenth and seventeenth centuries, when it was the greatest passion of the era. It was praised to the skies, and Shakespeare described it as "heavenly alchemy." It was known as the Royal Way; almost all the monarchs of Europe trod this path. In a painting by Jan Matejko the Polish alchemist Michał Sędziwój ("Sendivogius") is demonstrating transmutation to King Zygmunt III Wasa. How frail and fragile the king looks next to the famous alchemist, who emanates the power of his mysterious art. Is it any wonder that Sędziwój's work entitled *Novum Lumen Chymicum* would go through as many as fifty-four editions and would be plumbed to the depths by Isaac Newton?

The alchemists created an entire secret science, the *ars magna*, to obtain the elixir of life. We often imagine them in pursuit of gold, as precursors of the chemists who tried to change other substances into gold. But this image gives us only appearances and merely allows us to skim the surface of the matter, because alchemy "posed as a sacred science, whereas chemistry came into its own when substances had shed their sacred attributes."

As noted by Mircea Eliade, there was a striking similarity between alchemy and mining and metallurgy. "Very early on we are confronted with the notion that ores 'grow' in the belly of the earth after the manner of embryos. Metallurgy thus takes on the character of obstetrics." The miner and the metallurgist interfere in the course of this underground maturation and speed up the ores' rhythm of development, helping Mother Nature to give birth earlier. Just like the alchemist, thanks to the art they have mastered, they do Time's job for it by perfecting matter and completing its transmutation. In alchemy, transmutation was supposed to take place in several stages, two of which were defined by the names of colors: the black and the white.

For the alchemist, the first and most important step toward obtaining a perfect metal was to reduce a substance to its *materia prima*, or *massa confusa*, which corresponded on a cosmological level to the primeval state of being, that is, to chaos. This initial operation involved transformation into an amorphous state, through dissolution in mercury or carbonization by fire. Thus, it was a *regressus ad uterum*, a return to the prenatal stage. The *vas mirabile* (the furnace), which was supposed to contain the secret of alchemy, was like the womb (the uterus) that gave birth to the miraculous stone. At the very start of the operation there was blackness (the *nigredo*)—death as the initiator. It was impossible to achieve transmutation by starting from forms that had been used up by Time. First one had to dissolve them, so that later, by means of ablution, one could reach whiteness, which was the stamp of a successful result for the first part of the *opus magnum*.

A "work in white" (*leukosis* or *albedo*) following the *nigredo* corresponded on the spiritual level to resurrection, a new consciousness that was inaccessible to a worldly form. The art of transmutation is contained within the formula *solve et coagula* (cleanse and fuse). In coagulation the chemical and spiritual transformation fused together: dissolve everything that is inferior within you, then use the power achieved to solidify. For there is no doubt that by working to perfect matter, the alchemists were striving toward their own perfection. "Transform yourselves from dead stones into living philosophic stones!" we read in detailed descriptions of the experiments, while the *opus alchymicum* reveals profound analogies with mystical life. In their ovens, retorts, and *vas mirabile*, substances died and returned to their primeval chaos, in order to be resurrected and ultimately change into gold. The return to the womb, which both Chinese and Western alchemists wrote about, was a form of healing through a symbolic return to the source of origin, a recreation of the cosmogony. Many ancient therapies included a ritual reenactment of the creation of the world, allowing the patient to be born anew and start life over again. There was a firm belief that in this way it was possible to cure a man of being used up by Time, that is, of old age and death. And what about the actual Philosopher's Stone? Writing in the fifteenth century John Ripley, a master of the *ars magna*, said: "The birds and fishes bring the Stone to us, each man possesses it, it is everywhere, in you, in me, in all things, in time and in space. It is in all things created by God."

The attraction of alchemy must have been irresistible if it captivated even Isaac Newton. He practiced the *ars magna* night after night for many a long year, even when he was busy discovering that other force of attraction that rules the universe—gravity. These persistent attempts to transmute matter and soul, from the inferior to the superior, from the transient to the permanent, seemed to contain the conviction that once upon a time immortality was our privilege, and that all the arcane mysteries of alchemy tended to some extent toward finding a way back. As if original sin were, in the words of Czesław Miłosz, "just a Promethean dream about man, / a being so gifted that by the very force of his mind / he would create civilization and invent a cure for death."

What other paths could one take? A pact with the Prince of Darkness, following Faust's example, or placating the gods, something the Greeks knew all about. They had the chance to learn about it in ancient times, when the gods were happy to descend from Olympus to Earth. They were fond of amusing themselves there, undergoing metamorphoses, and making love. The Homeric heroes lived in close intimacy with them, without failing to keep the right distance. They had beauty, strength, and charm equal to that of the gods. They differed only in one respect: they lacked that inexhaustible spontaneity expressed in the gods' "inextinguishable laughter" (*asbestos gelos*), their ability to live without cares, "granted only to those few beings who are aware that they shall live without end."

Life without end is not everything, however. To be desirable, it has to be combined with eternal youth. Otherwise we might meet the fate of the Sibyl of Cumae. She is the only one of the five Sibyls on the ceiling of the Sistine Chapel to whom Michelangelo gave an old face, furrowed with wrinkles and anxiety. In her youth she asked Apollo for immortality, requesting as many years of life as the number of grains of sand she was able to hold in her hands. Once the request had been fulfilled, she refused Apollo the reward she had promised—her body—and so he punished her. In her request for eternal or incredibly long life she forgot to add that she wished to preserve her youth and beauty unimpaired. With the passage of time she grew older, becoming more and more shriveled, until in the end the priests put her in a little bottle and hung it on the wall. Whenever passing wayfarers asked her, "What is your desire, O Sibyl?" she answered, "I want to die."

Is it possible to remove someone from Time, to keep him as he is and protect him against change? Take the doctor's visit. I go up to a patient's bed. I realize that she is blind. I sit down beside her, take her hand and introduce myself.

"Ah, it's you, Doctor," she says. "I remember you so vividly, young and smiling."

"That must have been a long time ago," I say.

"Twenty-five years ago," she replies. "When I could still see and I was lying here in this hospital. To me, you have stayed just as you ever were. Time can't change that."

Some people used to say that Asclepius was not turned to ashes when struck by Zeus's thunderbolt, but that Apollo managed to change him into a snake in time. Apparently he lived for an extremely long time, watching over the history of medicine. What would he say about the practices of modern doctors? About their attempts to resuscitate victims of sudden death, for which he, Asclepius, paid the highest penalty?

In heart diseases death often comes suddenly. Sometimes bad news can kill a person. Sometimes violent changes in the weather, such as a *föhn* (an alpine wind), can kill. Sometimes it's physical overexertion. But in most cases we are unable to determine the trigger factor. The direct, precedent cause remains elusive. Nor does the time of day have a role to play, but dying at night, in one's sleep, is not a rare event. This unexpectedness is the hallmark of sudden death, and deprives it of the pathos of suffering, the struggle against illness, the fight for life. Its elements of surprise and speed cause amazement and fear in those left behind, reminding them how helpless they are in the face of blind, incomprehensible fate.

There are two ways for the heart to stop. In one, the ventricles stop working altogether. In the other the muscle fibers vibrate faintly and irregularly, so quickly and lightly that we call it ventricular fibrillation. Either way, the results are the same: the heart's pumping action stops, and not a single drop of blood is sent into circulation. An electrocardiogram allows us to distinguish these two forms of death.

Long before the electrocardiogram was invented, however, people tried to resuscitate the dead. There were lots of methods, ranging from flogging the dead with wicker canes to pull them from a state resembling far too deep sleep, or rubbing them with a mixture of herbs and fur shed by animals, to using a blacksmith's bellows to blow air into their lungs. In hospitals, especially in operating theaters, they also used to use "direct" heart massage: after hurriedly cutting the rib cage open and exposing the heart the doctor would squeeze it manually, causing blood to flow from the heart into the arteries.

At the beginning of the 1960s physicians discovered that it was just as effective to massage the heart and pump blood out of it without opening the rib cage. All you had to do was to rest the patient's back on a hard, solid surface, such as a board or a floor, and then place rhythmic pressure on the breastbone, a very flexible bone that passes the pressure on to the heart, which is immobilized from behind by the spine. Blood is rhythmically squeezed out of the heart and starts to circulate in the vessels again. When the heart stops, so does the breathing. It is therefore essential to apply artificial respiration. In the first instance, before the ambulance arrives, the lifesaver can pump air from his own lungs into those of the victim using the mouth-to-mouth method.

Learning the basic principles of resuscitation is already standard in elementary schools, state institutions, and civic organizations, not because there aren't enough doctors, but because time is of the essence. For a resuscitation attempt to have any chance of success, it must be started within three minutes. After that, irreversible changes start to happen in the brain.

No other illness results in sudden death as often as heart disease. Man has had to look that sort of death in the eye and has issued it a challenge. He has marked out an arena for the fight involved, and has named it the ICU—the intensive care unit. There he has stood his ground, armed with the most ingenious medical apparatus and some potent drugs. He has learned to listen for the steps of approaching death in his patients' hearts, and to seek the signs of its onset on electrocardiograms. He has come to recognize a few harbingers, which has sometimes enabled him to avert the seemingly inevitable end. In his audacity he has come such a long way that, surrounded by shining, luminous machinery, shielded by electronics, he has ventured onto terrain from which there had never been any way back until now. He has attempted to snatch back from death people whom it has already claimed and return sudden-death victims to life. He has proved that it is sometimes possible, although the competence, skill, and persistence of the doctors and nurses are more important factors than even the most sophisticated piece of equipment.

Conversations with patients who have survived clinical death and been saved do not usually tell us anything of substance. They are not able to say what happened to them, or to describe how it felt to be "on the other side." Their impressions, if they have any, seem to dissipate, just like even the most vivid of dreams the moment the dreamer wakes up. There's nothing left in the memory. The only people who remember anything are the ones who did the lifesaving. Their memories give them new energy for next time and allow them to entertain the hope that "maybe it'll work this time too?"

If it is possible to restore life, then why shouldn't old age cease to be inevitable? Cells collected from an embryo, cloned outside the organism and correctly programmed, will generate new tissue, whole new organs, even. Injected growth agents will retune an organism into a state of permanent regeneration. One day we may succeed in excluding the genes for old age from the embryo, making it quasi-immortal. We do not know when such techniques will become available and safe, but some scientists believe that it will happen. Scientific advances could extend the life span far beyond the age described as

> . . . second childishness and mere oblivion,
> Sans teeth, sans eyes, sans taste, sans every thing.

The human life span has already been extended by an incredible amount in the twentieth century. In the United States in 1900 it averaged forty-six years, and in 2000 seventy years. About twenty-five years of life added in a single century! The figures are similar for many Western European countries. As far as longevity goes, the best place to be born is Japan. At the beginning of the twenty-first century the average life span of a healthy person in Japan is seventy-four years (seventy-seven for women and seventy-two for men). Right behind it come Australia, France, Sweden, Spain, Italy, and Greece. Poland comes in sixty-first place, with an average of sixty-six years, but in Nigeria or Sierra Leone, placed 190th and 191st, the figures are only twenty-nine and twenty-five years, respectively.

Is there a gene that guarantees longevity or protects us against old age? A group of scientists in Boston has founded a commercial firm that screens the genes of sprightly old people in search of the one that guarantees them at least ninety years of life. The greatest hopes are focused on the telomer. If we imagine DNA as being like a shoelace, the telomer is the tag at each end. It is imperceptibly abraded every time the DNA comes unlaced in order to duplicate or transcribe itself. After years of "unlacing and lacing up again" the tag weakens and the shoelace becomes frayed and wears out. In an eighty-year-old the length of the telomer is getting dangerously short: it is half as long as it was at birth.

Our organism has its own system for repairing the telomer, involving its renovation, which can be done by an enzyme called telomerase. However, telomerase is a dormant knight in shining armor. It is only awake in the reproductive cells, in the life of an embryo. After that it falls into a permanent slumber. If only we could awaken it for good! If aging cells from human skin, in which the telomerase has been activated, are grafted onto a mouse, they behave like juveniles, full of energy and youth. Thus, telomerase is known as the "youth gene" and the "elixir of a cell's eternal life." And therefore the Boston scientists are looking for a way to regenerate it. There can be no doubt that telomerase prolongs the life of an individual cell toward the borders of immortality. But could it be done with an entire human being too? The skeptics are concerned that this is a dangerous path that will lead the cell onto the path of continual division — that is, toward cancer.

The newspapers recently published a photo of the deceased Frenchwoman Jeanne Clement of Arles. At 120 years old, she was the longest-living woman in the world, according to reliable registers. When I showed a color picture of her to my extremely elderly aunt, she bridled up and said: "Oh, no thank you very much!"

Women are thought to find it especially hard to bear the sight of their vanishing beauty, but men are not free of this fear either. Dorian Gray, the eponymous hero of Oscar Wilde's only novel, gazed with ever-greater shock at his portrait from the days of his innocent youth, which had the magical power of showing him his real face, which those around him couldn't see—until finally he stabbed the picture with a dagger.

The reaction of one of my patients to his own aging was also moving, though expressed in a different way. For a few days after being brought to the hospital by ambulance he was confused and depressed. Then he started to come back to us. When I came to see him I noticed how carefully he kept looking at himself in a small mirror. The next time I came he was clearly waiting to show me something. It was some old family photographs from ninety-one years ago. They showed a couple in their Sunday best, with their four small children. "The second from the right is me," said our patient, proudly showing me. "And this is me, and this too," he said, quickly extracting more photos from under the bedcovers. It was indeed him, in childhood, but not the second childhood now reflected in the mirror.

For thousands of years man's span of existence has continued to be invariable. Its range is demarcated, and those who have tried to overstep its bounds have been consumed by fire.

But we have increased the bounds of our existence. We have lengthened our life span. We have postponed death by decades. If it comes unexpectedly early, we do not hesitate to seize back its victims and restore them to life. But that is not the end of it. We are aiming to go much further. We are considering ways of creating humans, from a single cell. To avoid profanity, we talk of cloning. Is this the natural development of the Great Myth, or is it a form of denaturalization?

Let's take a look at the basic nature of medicine, the essence of this profession. It involves an encounter between two people, the patient and the doctor. In response to the patient's call for help, the doctor usually answers not in words, but with a smile or a gesture that says: "I'll stand by you. I won't desert you. Together we shall look mortal danger in the face." Answering the patient's call for help is the doctor's calling. And that's where myth enters into that encounter between two people. The doctor and the patient begin to share the same, primeval dream, and together they set out in search of the elixir of life.

IV. A TANGLE
OF SERPENTS

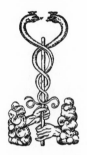

The simple Greeks rejected the poetic legend of Asclepius's death and believed that he went on living deep in the earth as a serpent endowed with great wisdom and human speech. Snakes became regular residents in the temples of Asclepius, which were run by doctors. These doctors were known as "asclepiads," the descendants of the god of medicine, a term which has survived to the present in the Polish language, where the word *eskulap* is a comic name for a doctor.

The temples of Asclepius were situated outside town, in the hills, among groves of trees and near springwater. The sick man who crossed the threshold of the temple underwent fasts and baths, put on a white robe, and made a propitiatory sacrifice (in later years it was a cockerel). The Greeks called these rituals the *katharmos*. They were supposed to purge one of guilt and unite one with the divinity. Next, "amid the silence and gloom of the temple, where tame snakes were coiled in every corner, the sick man fell into a prophetic dream." The priest-doctor appeared at night, dressed as Asclepius, with a retinue of helpers and servants,

and a snake. They went from patient to patient, in a procession re-
markably like the one that has done the rounds of our hospital
wards day in, day out, for centuries. We follow in their footsteps
and recreate their motions. The same is true of the act of healing,
which they performed at night, by symbolically laying on their
hands, administering medicine, or performing surgical operations. Early in the morning, after the nocturnal visit, the patient
woke up free of illness (having undergone *katharsis*) and healthy.
Sometimes the treatment took several nights, and its course was
influenced by the dreams the patient told the priests about. Some
of these dreams were recorded for posterity in the *Sacred Tales* of
Aelius Aristides and in thanksgiving votive offerings depicted on
the walls of the sanctuaries at Epidaurus, Pergamum, Lebena, and
Rome. The Greeks were fascinated by dreams. They sorted them
by category, analyzed them, and wrote them down. Thus, dream-
books have been written from the ancient Greek era right up to
our own times.

Children were brought to the temples too. The infant Cassan-
dra and her brother Helenus were left in the temple for the night,
and the next morning they were found entangled in the coils of
serpents, who by licking their eyes and ears had given them second sight and second hearing, a gift that gave them the power to
look into the future as easily as the present.

The serpent has been associated with Asclepius ever since. It
winds around his stick, and is thus a symbol of the medical profession, and also appears with the scales as a symbol of pharmacy.
By casting off its epidermis each year, the snake symbolizes regeneration. Its change of skin made a very strong impression on the
ancients. Philon of Alexandria believed it was the snake's way of
evading old age. He also credited it with the gifts of healing and
killing, and thus with the opposing forces that rule the world. The
synthesis of these contrasting forces is powerfully expressed in the
image of the feathered serpent, the most important symbol of

pre-Columbian America. It has feathers on its head and tail, sometimes on its entire body, which it uses to bind heaven and earth together.

The combination of a serpent and a stick has its ultimate expression in the Bible, where we read: "The Lord said to Moses, 'What is that in your hand?' He said, 'A staff.' And He said, 'Throw it on the ground.' So he threw it on the ground, and it became a serpent, and Moses ran from it. But the Lord said to Moses, 'Put out your hand and catch it by the tail.' So he put out his hand and caught it, and it became a staff in his hand."

When Moses struck the staff twice against a rock, a spring gushed from it, so what he had in his hand was a wand with secret powers. Since time immemorial the stick has been associated with magic. It was a mythical enchanted object, with the power to work miracles. We see it in the hand of the sorceress Circe, before her and after her, waved by the good fairy, who uses it to change a pumpkin into a carriage, and turns the wicked queen into a toad. "He who holds Prospero's magic stick in his hand, is the ruler—on STAGE," wrote the great Polish dramatist and artist Stanisław Wyspiański. So why shouldn't it be found in the hand of the god of medicine—an art derived from magic?

The caduceus, the wand of Hermes, whom the Romans called Mercury, has two snakes entwined around it. At their upper end they have small wings, sometimes a winged helmet too. The ancients ascribed magical power to the caduceus, which supposedly changed everything it touched to gold. Thus, it anticipated alchemy, and thousands of years later it was the alchemists who, through their refined analyses, made the furthest advances in analyzing the archetype of Mercury, herald of the gods. They identified him with the concept of flux and transformation. Mercury was said to possess an unlimited capacity for changing shape and came to personify the alchemists' desires—to transmute matter and spirit from the lower to the higher, from the transient to the permanent.

The two serpents entwined around the caduceus contained this power. They were an ancient symbol, originating from India and Mesopotamia at least three thousand years before Christ. The Mesopotamians regarded them as the image of a god healing sickness: the two S shapes created by the snakes were believed to correspond to sickness and convalescence. The way the two snakes contrast with each other signifies a balance of strengths. This frequently recurring image conceals a mystery: the snake is the omen and hallmark of sickness and at the same time its cure. The serpent heals the ailments caused by the serpent, and so within the illness itself lies the secret of its cure. Maybe that is why the Greek mind brought about an abstraction, and instead of the two primeval serpents that twined around the caduceus, we see only one now, on Asclepius's stick.

When in the year 293 BC their city suffered a plague epidemic, the Romans consulted the Sibylline Books, which were kept safe by a special college of curators. This was the ultimate step, decided upon only in extraordinary circumstances. The books told them to bring a sacred serpent from Epidaurus to Rome. It arrived by ship and went to live on an island in the river Tiber. We can have no doubt how the fate of the epidemic developed from then on, though history is silent on this point.

In the serpent, the commonplace was united with the mysterious. The paths wandered by its thoughts seemed completely different from those of people, just as the serpentine and human ways of moving about are different. What could be more peculiar than a snake—a creature with no arms or legs, no eyelids, ears, or voice, yet which is fearless, agile, completely still or fast as lightning, hissing, independent and as a rule solitary, and capable of inflicting death by strangulation in its embrace or a poisonous bite. The snake caught man in its spell, and man took it into his world of charms, making it the symbol of primeval cosmic forces, divine influence, healing powers, autogenesis, rejuvenation, sensuality and fertility, cunning and intelligence.

The Pharaohs wore it on their foreheads: Ureus, the symbol of their power, was represented by an attacking cobra, sometimes winged and breathing fire. However, the Greeks and Romans regarded snakes as the guardian spirits of the temple, and often kept them as domestic pets to get rid of rats and mice. "The children would play with snakes, and ladies used them to cool their necks and chests in summer." In ancient Greece, as in India, they were believed to bring good luck and were a talisman against the forces of evil. In other mythologies the idea of eternal enmity between snakes and people was extremely rare. It was not until the book of Genesis that a gulf appeared, separating snake and man. "I will put enmity between you and the woman, and between your offspring and her offspring; he shall bruise your head, and you shall bruise his heel." And since then, forevermore that "narrow Fellow," who without warning "in the grass occasionally rides," evokes just one reaction in us:

> But never met this Fellow
> Attended, or alone
> Without a tighter breathing
> And Zero at the Bone—

Dreams and serpents made a comeback several thousand years later . . . to lay the foundations for organic chemistry. In the mid-nineteenth century it was known that benzene consists of six carbon atoms linked with six hydrogen atoms. C_6H_6—what a simple formula! The only problem was that no one could begin to imagine how the carbon atoms were spatially connected. They were arranged in a chain, like people holding hands, but those hands, corresponding to chemical bonds, did not add up. At one point it would have been better to have more of them, at another fewer, and the ones at each end of the open chain were empty. Then August Kekulé imagined the chain closed to form a ring, and it all made sense. That first, simple, ring-shaped structure started off an enormous family of cyclic compounds of carbon.

We come across them everywhere in nature, and they even make up the letters of the genetic code.

Twenty-five years after describing the cyclical structure of benzene, Kekulé attended a grand ceremony in Berlin, where he told how he had seen the solution to the enigma of benzene in a dream.

Apparently it happened toward evening by a bonfire near Ghent. As the twisting tongues of flame grew more and more like snakes, Kekulé fell asleep. Then a single snake separated itself from the forest of flaming serpents, seized its own tail as if trying to swallow it, and closed itself off in the form of a ring. The ring—that was the solution. Before Kekulé saw it, the serpent devouring its own tail had been seen by the ancient Greeks, before them by the Egyptians, and even earlier by the Sumerians. It was Ouroboros, who constantly devours himself and regenerates, never vanishes, but is always changing in an eternal cycle of destruction and rebirth.

Kekulé was accused of making up the story after the fact. But he had actually located his dazzling discovery within mythological reality, in a dream dreamed by man since the beginning of time.

The serpent has always represented the opposing forces of killing and healing. This notion has been corroborated in the past few decades, when snake venom, which has deprived so many people of life, has also helped us to discover some extremely effective medicines.

In the mid-1960s a Brazilian research student called Sergio Ferreira turned up at the London laboratory of pharmacologist John Vane, who later won the Nobel Prize. He did not hide the fact that he was there by accident—he had come on a scholarship to Oxford, but his wife wanted to do her PhD at the London School of Economics, which was near Vane's laboratory. So he stayed on, and soon every corner of the lab was filled with his loud, infectious laughter and his aromatic cigar smoke. Quite casually, pretty much carrying it in his pocket, he had brought along an extract from the venom of a poisonous snake, *Bothrops jararaca,* whose properties he had been researching in Brazil. Thanks to the bioassay, an original experimental technique developed by Vane, his team proved that the extract brought by Sergio could block the activity of an enzyme called convertase. This enzyme produces a substance in the lungs that causes extreme constriction of the arteries. John Vane noticed that the venom could be used as the embryo of a drug to counteract high blood pressure. He persuaded Squibb, the large American pharmaceutical firm, to isolate the active substance from the snake venom, which turned out to be a short peptide, consisting of nine amino acids. Applied intravenously to patients suffering from hypertension, it brought their blood pressure down. Shortly after, analogues and derivatives of this peptide were synthetized and introduced in the form of an oral drug. And thus a new class of drugs for hypertension was born: convertase inhibitors. The first two drugs (captopril and enalapril) achieved annual sales worth millions of dollars. Nowadays there are at least ten other convertase inhibitors on the market, available in a huge number of forms, under various trade names.

Sergio Ferreira was not the first person to bring snake venom to London with him. Forty years before him an Australian called Charles Kellaway sailed from Melbourne to London on a research scholarship, taking some test tubes full of cobra venom on the journey. He knew that the cobra's bite led to suffocation and shock. In London he injected the snake venom into the isolated lungs of a guinea pig and discovered that it caused the release of a substance that greatly constricted the bronchi. This same substance, produced by the lungs and liberated by the snake venom, was later found to appear in the human airways during asthma attacks and anaphylactic shock, but getting hold of it had proved almost impossible, because it vanished in a matter of seconds. Ingenious chemical traps had been set for it, but with no success. The first person to capture it was Bengt Samuelsson, who proved that the mystery substance was a mixture of compounds whose structure he defined and named leukotrienes. In 1979 at a congress in Washington, DC, Samuelsson disclosed the chemical structure of leukotrienes. The next day the front page of every American newspaper carried the headline: "The Riddle of Asthma Has Been Solved." Three years later Bengt Samuelsson and John Vane were awarded the Nobel Prize for their joint work in this sphere. However, twenty years had to pass before drugs blocking leukotrienes were brought into practice. They are a valuable weapon in treating asthma, but we are still a long way from solving the riddle of this disease.

In myth, primeval serpents are the world's mainstay, providing it with matter and energy. And when Zeus reached back in his memory, he returned to the years preceding his father, Chronos, then withdrew further and further into the depths of time, and finally stopped at the point "that was furthest, because it had been the first.

"Space no longer existed. In its place was a convex surface clad with thousands upon thousand of scales. It extended beyond anything the eye could see. Looking downward along the scales, he realized that they were attached to other scales, the same color, interwoven with them in knot after knot, each one tighter than the one before. The eye became confused, could no longer tell which of the two coiling bodies the scales belonged to. As he looked up again, toward the heads of the two knotted snakes, the body of the first snake rose, and its scales merged into something that no longer partook of the nature of a snake: it was the face of a god. . . .

"From the shoulders opened immense, airy wings. The white arm of a woman was twined to the arm of the god, just as below the tails of the two snakes were knotted together. The woman's face gazed steadily at the god's, while with her other arm, behind which trembled an immense wing, she stretched out toward the farthest extremity of everything: and where the tips of her fingernails reached, there Everything ended. They were a royal and motionless couple: they were Time-without-Age and Ananke."

In the nucleus of every one of the billions of cells in our bodies deoxyribonucleic acid, or DNA, lies hidden. It has the shape of a double, serpentine spiral and contains the secret of life's regeneration. It lies within us as a memory, a vestige, a reflection of the royal couple of snakes from whose union the world was born.

V. IN BETWEEN ART
AND SCIENCE

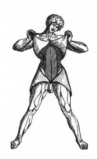

If illness is "a confession of the body," doctors have made every effort to plumb its depths and find the cause of the illness—to see what lies hidden inside man. In Alexandria in the third century BC corpses were routinely dissected. The Egyptian rulers were so keen on supporting science that they handed criminals over to learned doctors for vivisection, enabling them to see inside the body of a living man: "the color, shape, size, structure, hardness, softness and smoothness of every organ; what it adjoins, where it bulges and where it sinks, where it attaches and what it covers," as Celsus wrote about it several centuries later, with some envy, as by then dissection was prohibited. Galen of Pergamum (129–216 AD) claimed "to have performed a dissection every day for most of his working life," exercising the manual dexterity that is crucial to a surgeon, and getting to know the innermost secrets of the body. He looked inside all sorts of animals, including the emperor's pet elephant, but he never touched a human corpse, because it was against the law.

But it was the great anatomist Andreas Vesalius of Padua who first revealed the world locked inside us in his famous *De humani corporis fabrica*. This seven-volume work aroused universal admiration for its erudition and editorial standard; the illustrations were done by Renaissance masters, mainly from the school of Titian. Three hundred and fifty years later the father of American medicine, Dr. William Osler, called Vesalius's work "the greatest book in medicine."

But how much Vesalius must have had to go through to produce it! In his memoirs he describes how he used to steal corpses from graveyards to complete skeletons, fighting off savage dogs as he did so. He encouraged his students to familiarize themselves with the details of the illnesses that their professors' patients were suffering from, in order to seize their bodies as soon as they died. In embittered moments he wrote: "I shall not keep in my bedroom for several weeks bodies taken from graves or given me after public execution." Thus, he was like Hans Holbein the Younger, when he painted that long, narrow, life-size portrait of Christ lying on his back, tortured to death. In Dostoyevsky's *The Idiot* Prince Myshkin says that looking at that painting could make you lose your faith, because "that corpse would never rise from the dead." Apparently when he painted it, Holbein borrowed a corpse from the city guard for a small fee; he returned it at daybreak after a night spent painting, face to face with death.

Vesalius performed all his dissections himself, in which regard he was an exception. Until then they were done by a barber, while the professor, sitting at a distance from the corpse, read aloud from Galen's notes, written fifteen centuries earlier, mainly on the anatomy of monkeys and dogs, which the great Roman doctor rather blithely transferred to man. Do I need to add that in Vesalius's time there was no such thing as protective gloves or antiseptic?

A hundred years later, Rembrandt painted two anatomy lessons. The first was a commission for the surgeons' guild, which he received as a young man. In the picture Dr. Nicolaes Tulp, *praelector anatomiae,* Amsterdam's foremost demonstrator of anatomy, is revealing the muscles and tendons of the forearm that make the fingers bend. This action copies the gesture of Vesalius as depicted in a painting by Stephan van Calcar. Calm and concentrated, in his right hand he is holding up the tendons of the hand, gripped in a forceps, to show them to the students of surgery. Extremely moved, they are leaping out of their seats to avoid missing anything. This vivid scene, dramatically lit, brought Rembrandt success and further commissions. But there were also those who carped that he had not started the autopsy by opening the belly, which was the usual practice, and they whispered that maybe he had never actually attended a dissection. Twenty-five years later they got their answer.

In 1656 Rembrandt painted an anatomy lesson given by Dr. Johan Deyman, who was Dr. Tulp's successor. The picture was damaged by fire in the eighteenth century. As you look at it nowadays in the Rijksmuseum, you might think it was ignited by its own inner ardor. Seen from below, the corpse goes off the edge of the picture. The soles of its feet are pointed at the viewer, and there is a gaping hole in its empty belly, like Rembrandt's slaughtered ox in the Louvre or the Budapest art gallery. Its raised head stares toward us. The master is not fully visible, just his hands on the dead man's exposed brain. To the side an assistant, dressed in black, with a white, turned-down collar and his hair hanging loose, is holding the top of the skull, turned upside down like a bowl. This inherently repellent object has been transformed into a painter's vision, changed into a mysterious, splendid show of color and light, a scene dominated by the dead man's head, to which "death has lent shockingly large dimensions."

How wonderful to admit a ray of light into the darkness locked in the body forever, to open it up and see inside! However, not everything was instantly visible. Even the great Vesalius overlooked the pancreas, the ovaries, and the adrenal glands and did not make a very good job of depicting the uterus. But then he had to leave something for his illustrious pupils to do. And with their vision reinforced by the lenses of microscopes, their successors set about investigating the delicate structures of the organs, invisible to the naked eye. Others sought the vestiges of illness in them. And so the edifice of anatomy was built—descriptive, pathological, and forensic—the *theatrum anatomicum,* on the stage of which the last judgment of illness was held, a judgment with no opportunity for appeal. Such was the edifice of anatomy on 14 August 1944 in Danzig where, in Stefan Chwin's novel *Death in Danzig,* in a spacious dissection room the students "silently grouped around the marble slab table," waited with rising tension for the entry of Professor Hanemann, fetched from home in a black Daimler-Benz sent specially for him, so that he might unravel the mystery of the death of a young woman fished out by the pier at Glettkau, where the small excursion boat *Stern* had sunk. Anatomy was just the same in the decades that followed and when I was a student, acting as the final verification of a clinical diagnosis. But with the passage of time, tentatively at first, then more and more boldly and vigorously, doctors have started collecting samples of tissues and organs from their patients, using a careful eye to prod whatever possible, wherever they can reach with a needle. And body samples of this kind, taken from the living, have been used to open up a picture of the illness without waiting to open the entire body after death. The burden of final diagnosis has begun to shift elsewhere. But anatomy—more and more neglected—has stayed at a standstill in its increasing, royal solitude.

Have the unquenchable curiosity and passion of Vesalius and his successors, or the permanent edifices of anatomy, physiology, microbiology, and pharmacology, caused medicine to become a science? No, is the staunch reply of the eminent physicist Andrzej Białas. To elaborate his argument, he quotes a remark made seventy years ago by his great colleague Ernest Rutherford: "All science is either physics or stamp collecting." To which one could jokingly reply in the words of another eminent physicist, Andrzej Staruszkiewicz, who says: "In those days the physicists were in a really good mood." Yet the question is not trivial, and from Rutherford's perspective it should be formulated: Does medicine stand a chance of ever becoming physics? In other words, of quantitatively defining the phenomena it observes and producing a precise, mathematical image of reality? Despite the staggering achievements of medicine we are not aware of any laws governing the human body, in sickness or in health, which we could encapsulate in mathematical equations. Does a doctor ever go looking for the sort of mathematical formulas that are prototypical for physical objects—even the ones that are all around him on a daily basis? Does he ever try to guess the mathematical construction of physical reality, which there is no way of inferring from pure observation? Universal in theoretical physics, this sort of "identification" principle is unknown to medicine. Was it that medical and mathematical learning repelled each other and refused to live together inside the same skull? I think not—the complexity of the subject is a more likely explanation.

Modern physics came into being when Galileo and others said: "Understanding how the entire world works is incredibly difficult, so meanwhile let's try to get to know a given phenomenon in isolation from everything else. Let's try to understand how a stone falls from a leaning tower." This method, known as reductionism because it endeavors to reduce complex phenomena to a combination of a certain number of elementary ones, has brought spectacular results. Many physicists reckon we are on the eve of fulfilling the dream of the ancients: to construct a "theory of everything."

Perhaps none of the early thoughts of the great Greek philosophers was more admirable than the idea that variable phenomena have a constant nature. Anaximander reflected on the *arche*—the permanent, primeval nature of things. Parmenides propounded the leading theory of the unity and invariability of existence. Empedocles set about searching for the simple components of matter and can be regarded as the creator of the concept of the elements. And finally Democritus established a theory that held that matter is composed of atoms. "They are unchanging, but they move about in space and create a changing, ever-different structure for the world."

Is one single "theory of everything" possible, as considered by the Greeks, and which has had a modern revival—a perfect theory of matter that would cover all the elementary particles, fields, and energies and link them with the origin of the universe? The great physicists have always attempted to unify apparently discrete phenomena: Gallileo tried with terrestrial and celestial laws, Newton with gravity and the movement of celestial bodies, Maxwell with magnetism and electricity, and Einstein with space and time. Today's physicists are pinning their hopes for an explanation of the world's fundamental structure on the "superstring" theory. What makes it attractive is undoubtedly its elegance and its many symmetrical features. Throughout history scientists have been guided by aesthetic principles; the great English theoretical physicist Paul Dirac once said that it is more important for a theory to be beautiful than for it to match experience. Yet the superstring theory and its most recent amendments "provide only abstract images, which do not allow us to visualize the structure of atoms or the dynamics of space—time or the topology of the universe in any direct sense." Formulating a single "theory of everything" might be an impossible task for several reasons. Firstly, the quantum theory, the best of the scientific theories we have at our disposal, introduces an inherent element of uncertainty related to any measurement of a physical structure. Next there is the knotty problem of self-referentiality, arising from the fact that the measuring tools we use to study nature are part of it themselves. Finally there is the difficulty, or even the impossibility of explaining unique, individual phenomena, in other words the so-called origins problem. As science studies recurrent processes, there is much doubt whether questions about the origin of the universe or of life can be posed by science at all. Even mathematics, which is meant to be the language in which the laws of nature are written, teaches us that there are questions to which we cannot find the answers by applying its rules. Kurt Gödel demonstrated that in any coherent logical system there are theorems whose truth or falsehood cannot be determined. All this makes us aware of the limits of scientific knowledge.

Clinical medicine draws on the discoveries of biology, biochemistry, genetics, and pharmacology by the handful. It brings research laboratories under its roof and takes part in highly refined analyses of the patient's blood and tissues to disclose genes that are predisposed to an illness. It closely follows experiments on animals, looking for reflections of what goes on in a patient's body—all in order, at the decisive moment, to proceed with the only definitive experiment: on man himself.

In 1976, at the London laboratory of John Vane, in a flash of genius Ryszard Gryglewski discovered prostacyclin, a hormone produced by the lining of the arteries. We immediately realized that here in our hands we were holding something extremely interesting. But were we really holding it? Prostacyclin turned out to be a volatile, ephemeral substance that disintegrated after only a few seconds. It was possible to prove how the arteries produce it, but it was incredibly difficult to catch hold of it and keep it. To achieve its synthesis we turned to America for help. I remember the symposium in Chicago a few months later. Joseph Fried, one of their best chemists, gave a presentation. He showed us dozens of spatial combinations in which the fifty-six atoms that make up a prostacyclin molecule might be arranged. But which was the right one? The situation looked hopeless. Then Fried said: "From my calculations it appears that one of the structures whose pattern I have presented on the board has the greatest likelihood of existing. Prostacyclin can only be like this. I have synthesized it and brought it to show you." As he said this, he drew a tiny little test tube from his top pocket with a pinch of white powder at the bottom. Needless to say, we spent the night with Fried at the bar, and the next day we flew back to Poland with about a dozen milligrams of the priceless powder. Not everyone believed in Fried as we did, nor was everyone inclined to imagine that a powerful physiological and healing force might lie hidden in prostacyclin.

We were in a mad hurry. What was driving us? Curiosity, for sure, but also the sporting spirit that's always present in science: we wanted to be first. Patriotism too. For me, additionally, it was the joy of working with a friend.

Back in Cracow, quick as lightning we performed some experiments on cats to establish the dose of prostacyclin that a cat could tolerate. We converted the weight of a cat into our own, then took turns lying down in the intensive care unit at the hospital at 8 Skawińska Street. And that's how it began. After only a few minutes of intravenous infusion of prostacyclin Ryszard Gryglewski lost consciousness. The prostacyclin had dilated his blood vessels and had lowered his blood pressure to an indeterminable value. It took a while before we managed to bring him back to his senses. (We joked afterwards that the truly revelatory conclusion of our experiments was that a kilogram of cat is not the same as a kilogram of man!) When it was my turn and I was receiving prostacyclin, I began to shake with fever and my temperature rose to 41°C. The reason was simple. Despite the use of microbiological filters, during its dissolution the prostacyclin had become contaminated with bacteria, which I had injected along with it into my veins. When I got home, consumed by fever, I found my wife in the doorway with our small son in her arms, intent on leaving me for ever because I had broken my word and was still doing experiments on myself. It felt like an eternity before I had persuaded her to stay, and another eternity before I collapsed onto the couch, shivering with cold, pulled an eiderdown over myself, and on top of it a second, third, and fourth blanket.

After us, our colleagues at the hospital received intravenous infusions of prostacyclin without any complications. Once we had understood and described the powerful effect of prostacyclin on human blood circulation and clotting, we were soon using it to treat diseases of the peripheral arteries. We selected patients facing amputation of the limbs, for whom there was no longer any alternative. How many days and nights we spent at their bedsides, listening out for the piercing pain in their feet to quieten down, and not believing our own eyes when the deep ulcers on their shins shrank and dwindled as the blood was mixed with a daily dose of prostacyclin. After these initial successes we went through a phase of exaggerated hopes, expecting prostacyclin to be a panacea for common diseases of the heart and brain, which turned out to be completely untrue. Nowadays, years on, stable analogues of prostacyclin have an established position within the treatment of pulmonary hypertension, and also in treating arteriosclerosis and Bürger's disease, which attack distal sections of the arteries.

From these experiments on the entire organism it is time to return to the components of the human body. This is in keeping with the principle of reductionism: to understand how a machine works, you have to dismantle it, reducing it to its smallest parts. Reductionism has flourished in biology. Molecular biology—the driving force for the natural sciences—seems to be one big triumph of reductionism. We have deciphered the genetic code, recognized the sequence of three billion little letters; now all we have to do is skillfully put them together into words and sentences—and there we have the recipe for man! We are so fascinated by these truly staggering achievements that nowadays we tend to ascribe a greater role to the parts than the whole. Our genes are getting out of hand, becoming independent, and starting to play their own game of life. These "selfish genes" are fighting each other for survival in the chain of evolution. And although "the individual organism is not exactly an illusion," it is in fact "a secondary, derived phenomenon, cobbled together as a consequence of the action of fundamentally separate, warring agents." Ringing metaphors —like the "selfish gene" of the Oxford biologist and talented popularizer of science Richard Dawkins, or the "self-multiplying particle" of Francis Crick, the codiscoverer of DNA—exert a powerful influence on the outlook of biologists and medics. Yet DNA does not multiply all by itself. To do that it needs a lot of elements and mechanisms, all provided by the cell that encloses it. Moreover, genes are only about 2% of DNA. So what is the rest? We know almost nothing about it. It certainly isn't "junk," as some scientists have defined it. The problem we come up against in trying to understand how the expression of genes is regulated or in trying to find the genes responsible for common illnesses would seem to imply that we need a different, integrated outlook on the phenomena of life.

The stunning effectiveness of reductionism in physics, chemistry, or molecular biology is also attractive to other branches of knowledge, such as psychology. If only we could tame it and simplify our inner life, making it subject to the well-known principles of matter, so that it would stop causing us bother! Many people have sought the material foundations for this in neurology and evolutionism. There is an echo of the "selfish gene" in sociology, in the form of attempts to explain social phenomena by analyzing small communities and the behavior of individuals. But such "atomization of society," a term that reminds us Poles of the dreadful experience of martial law, has never yet fulfilled the hopes placed in it. Opponents of reductionism point out that the method is not only commonly applied in science, but also uncritically. And they illustrate their point with the joke about the man who goes looking for his keys at night under a lamppost; when asked if that's where he lost them, he replies: "Not at all, but it'll be the easiest place to find them!"

In the human body the organs are so greatly interconnected that applying something roughly like an "isolated system" to them seems dubious. We would have to go beyond "reductionism" and create a new method of researching these structures, which are difficult to break down into their constituent parts. In the language of mathematics we speak of "systems that cannot easily be brought closer through the linear superimposing of their simple elements." This means that certain structures cannot be obtained through the simple addition of their components. There are feedbacks at work within them: the individual parts have a mutual effect on one another. "The whole, considered in relation to its parts, contains a structural surplus," or as Aristotle said, "The whole is more than the sum of the parts." We are gradually getting to know the principles that govern these processes, which are called "nonlinear dynamical systems." They are already enabling us to observe turbulence or other critical phenomena, including catastrophe, and also to move away from simplified, deterministic interpretations of evolution—that of both galaxies and living organisms.

Research into nonlinear dynamical systems has become the central issue in physics. In these systems behavior that is most difficult to understand can arise from what would seem to be the most humble of origins. The simple principles lead to the emergence of complex structures. Complex phenomena in nature do not therefore necessarily result from compound laws of nature, but may arise from their nonlinearity. So could the principles that govern living organisms, including man, be so simple that they could be discovered, formulated, and recorded by the methods of physics? If it were ever to come to this, we would have no problem getting physicists to award medicine the status of a science.

Somewhere in between science and art, the doctor stands at a crossroads, because these two creative endeavors are usually regarded as opposites. "It is not for art / to seek truth that is the task of science," wrote Zbigniew Herbert. According to Henryk Elzenberg there is a clash between the scientific turn of mind and the evaluative kind of thinking typical of art that is hard to reconcile. Years later, Herbert, who was Elzenberg's pupil, made an oblique reference to his master's incisive remark by composing an apocryphal letter from the painter Jan Vermeer to a friend from Delft, the maker of the microscope, Antony van Leeuwenhoek. Science, writes Vermeer in Zbigniew Herbert's version, is meant "to give . . . certain, clear knowledge, which according to you is the only defense against fear and anxiety. But will it really bring us relief if we substitute the word *necessity* for the word *Providence*?" However, the duty of art is not "to solve enigmas, but to be aware of them, to bow our heads before them and also to prepare the eyes for never-ending delight and wonder." The "archaic procedure" of art relies on telling "the world words of reconciliation" and speaking of "joy from recovered harmony, of the eternal desire for reciprocated love."

Outside the hospital on Skawińska Street in Cracow, which for the final years of his life was a second home to the popular cabaret star Piotr Skrzynecki (he christened it "the Hotel of Dreams"), stands a sculpture dedicated to his memory. It features two acrobats, a man and a woman, balancing in defiance of the force of gravity. It reminds us of the wizardry of the Great Magus from the Piwnica pod Baranami cabaret, as well as the art of medicine, which balances on the border between life and death. Both have a common origin in magic. This particular origin of medicine is worth remembering nowadays, as it transforms itself into a science.

However, science is just one way of learning about reality.

Plato knew this, and as he came near the limits of scientific learning, he turned to poetry to take him across the border where reason was forced to turn back. Through poetic metaphors, through art, he captured truths that were inaccessible to science. But what, we might ask, is the truth? "The truth is a mobile army of metaphors," replies Friedrich Nietzsche. If this truth about the truth is true, then the circle closes, art meets up with science, and the doctor finds his place at the point where they connect.

VI. THE RHYTHM
OF THE HEART

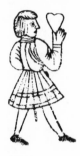

The world around us is overflowing with rhythms. We are always coming into contact with them, from the moment we are born. The rocking of the cradle and the singing that goes with it are both rhythms; so are the flash of a lighthouse beam and the roar of waves crashing against the shore, the rattle of a train and the croaking of frogs by the tracks. The world's rhythms pervade us, bringing in their own meter and stirring a response. Among primitive peoples rhythm is associated with the beginning of life. On the Polynesian islands a god molded a figurine of woman-as-the-mother out of clay and then danced before her for three days and three nights. Drums accelerated the rhythm, while with every movement of his dancing body he implored and incited her. Until finally—as Czesław Miłosz writes—matter could no longer maintain its own inertia. The first shudder of rhythm ran through the figurine, waking her from an ageless sleep. Her first response was shy: she stuck out one knee, testing to see if she were really made of something other than earth.

Or maybe the rhythm beaten out on the drums came from

deep inside the universe? Was it perhaps aroused by signals flowing from interstellar space, steady and regular, emerging from inside rapidly rotating colossi that make our sun look like a speck of dust? Known as neutron stars, these gigantic concentrations of matter, the sources of powerful magnetic and gravitational fields, send radio waves of great intensity into the universe—and to us as well. They are typically so perfectly regular that the centers where they arise are called pulsars. So is it impossible to imagine that the pulsars imposed their rhythm on the beating drums, and that the first pulse of blood that ran through man, stirring him into life, was a response to their rhythm? Was the human pulse set off by the pulsars of the universe?

It is not just the world that sends its rhythms coursing through us. There are also rhythms inside us. There are so many rhythmic processes happening in our bodies, from the obvious ones, like sleeping and waking, to the most well hidden, like the secretion of hormones into the blood, that to explain their uncanny regularity and synchronicity we have adopted the figurative idea of the biological clock. Long before it was discovered, everyone agreed that if this extraordinary chronometer really did exist, then every last cell of our bodies would be able to tell the time from it.

Nowadays we locate it in the brain, in the part called the hypothalamus. The biological clock runs in two concentrations of gray matter, known as the hypothalamic nuclei, and so does its most essential part—the circadian oscillator. The clock's mechanism appears to be determined by a cycle of recurring reactions: the transcription of genes and the synthesis of proteins. These reactions form a feedback loop: so-called clock genes code proteins, which accumulate and retroactively obstruct the transcription of genes. As protein disintegrates, transcription gets going again, and the protein production cycle is resumed. This "clockwork" system, characterized by rhythmicality, is common to all species, from the fruit fly to man. It is teamed with the emission of circadian signals, which depend on changes in the cell's membrane potential. Once in existence, they spread into the nearest vicinity and to other areas of the brain as well.

But what use would a watch be if you couldn't set it to local time? The biological clock is buried in the brain just above the intersection of the optic nerves. Converted light signals take a short cut to bring it a constant supply of information about the world, just as the neurons that make up its structure provide it with information from inside the body. Within the "clock-gene" mechanism the rhythms of the internal and external worlds converge and harmonize.

Some people's biological clock runs fast. At the dawn of the third millennium several families were identified in the state of Utah, all of whose members—from grandparents to grandchildren—wake up four hours earlier than everyone else. They leap out of bed feeling full of energy, while their neighbors remain fast asleep for some time to come. Their clock seems to be set four hours ahead. In these early birds there has been a change in a single little letter, a nucleotide in one of their clock genes. Or perhaps the "night owls" carry a different, subtle genetic mutation within their clock? Medicine is now starting to look for drugs that can interfere in the working of the biological clock, to correct the disagreeable jet lag that we experience after transatlantic flights, for example. Will a new kind of doctor emerge in the future . . . known as a "clockmaker"? Will the Polish minister of health have to add a new medical specialty to the current list of seventy-two? And to avoid confusion with clockmakers, will he give these specialists a scholarly name, "chronologists," for instance?

Of the many rhythms beating away inside our bodies the heartbeat is the one we care about most, perhaps because it has always been the hallmark of life—both biological and emotional. Doesn't the doctor listen to his patient's heartbeat just as attentively as the novelist listens to his hero's? Don't both of them borrow each other's words to describe the heart's condition, saying that it is throbbing, fluttering, or fading?

As far back as the longest-lasting consistent civilization ever to have existed, the world of ancient Egypt, the heart played an enormous role, as the center of psychological strength too. It comes into poetry, religion, and hieratic texts, and rises to the rank of not only the central organ in the body, but also the main seat of the emotions—virtually becoming "the essence of the essence" of man. In the era of the Old Kingdom, five thousand years ago, nothing but a man's heart would be tossed onto the scales at the posthumous judgment of Osiris. To be pure, a heart set on the scales before the god had to weigh less than the lightest feather. Otherwise, it was immediately gobbled up by a monster waiting by, and the Egyptian's life beyond the grave ended in eternal ignominy.

As for the heart, it's not so much its harmony with the rhythms of the surrounding world as its rhythm's independence that is its most amazing feature. Think back to our school biology lessons— if you remove a frog's heart and put it on the table top, it goes on beating for several long minutes. Every day in hundreds of operating theaters all over Europe surgeons stop a sick heart and cool down the body to perform complex operations, and once they've finished, they set the heart going again with an electric shock. During transplantation the heart taken from the donor's body is left on its own for several hours in a nourishing liquid that is simple to make; later on it ends up inside an organism that is alien to it, but once aroused by a current applied to its walls for a split second, it starts up a steady beat. These examples show that within the heart itself there must be a mechanism capable of setting it going rhythmically.

This mechanism is made up of specialized cells that generate and distribute impulses. They are not scattered at random, but are linked to form a compound structure. We call it the automatic system of the heart or, more often, the conductive system. The first name stresses the independence and above all the infallible, mechanical regularity with which the system works, and the second emphasizes the role it plays in dispersing the impulses. Large clusters of cells within the system form nodes, or stations, between which the impulses run along the tracks of fibers. Just like an army at the front, the conductive system has its own hierarchy, assuring that leadership is continually handed on in the event of the leader's death. At the top of the hierarchical ladder stands the sinoatrial, or sinus, node, which sets the pace, or takes the first step. It produces the highest-frequency impulses and thus stifles all the other potential pacemakers, dictating the rhythm of the entire heart. If it should become impaired, the role of leader is assumed by the next nodes down the hierarchy, successively setting rhythms of lower and lower frequency. When they too fall silent, the heart activates its emergency rescue mechanism, concealed in the muscle, and starts beating at the slowest rhythm that will guarantee a supply of blood to the organs at rest but will not allow for any effort at all. In such cases we speak of total heart block, as the intermediate stations and previously passable routes to them have been destroyed or obstructed.

What are the signals we have followed to make the journey from the first station right through to the last? We describe them as being electrical in nature, and we say that they come into being when fissures appear in the cell walls, tiny channels along which some charged atoms drop inside and others drop out. This event recurs rhythmically, causing potential differences. The electrical discharges travel along the routes familiar to us all the way to the muscle fibers, where they set off a contraction. But inside the cell walls, who opens the gate to such a precise rhythm, allowing the charged atoms to leap through in opposite directions? What sort of metronome beats out this primary rhythm, which sets the rhythm of the heart? We don't know the answer, and even with the idea of an electrical current we are skating over the surface of what actually occurs.

Do our hearts beat with the mechanical perfection of a metronome? Not everyone's does, as the following explanation shows. Impulses repeatedly continue to arise in the cells of the sinoatrial node to a perfect rhythm, like the beat of the most sensitive of metronomes. But before an impulse leaves the node, in order to disperse along the trails created for it and prompt the heart to contract, it experiences the extremely subtle influence of the sympathetic nervous system. This is a very delicate effect, which as a rule we are unable to detect with a stethoscope. However, we can perceive it by analyzing a long electrocardiogram recording. When we measure the gaps between consecutive heartbeats over a period of several minutes, we notice that in many of us there are tiny differences between them, and that they deviate from the average by hundredths of a second.

This reminds us of the musical tempo rubato, which is a typical feature of Chopin's work. There are lots of familiar definitions of Chopin's rubato. Some say it describes performing a composition "with a subtle rhythmic anxiety." Others say that rubato relies on "tiny shifts between the notes of the melody within the range of its own beat, against a steadily paced bass." Franz Liszt characterized Chopin's rubato by comparing it to a tree, "when its crown bends in all directions in the wind, but its roots are stuck firmly in the ground."

Chopin used the term *rubato* to denote playing *senzo rigore* in his mazurkas and nocturnes written in the years 1824–1835, but from 1836 he stopped using it. According to Gastone Belotti the reasons for this are obvious: as soon as he reached maturity all his compositions were to be played rubato.

There are some hearts in which the rubato, that "subtle rhythmic anxiety," clearly registers, as in Chopin's mature work, and there are others in which—as in his earlier, youthful work—it is not perceptible. When struck by a dangerous illness, the former are less likely to stop suddenly, as if a lack of stiffness, a sort of flexibility, or a tendency toward a free and easy beat had prepared them better for the onset of malevolent, morbid rhythms. Analysis of these discreet deviations from the perfect rhythm under the influence of the nervous system (known as "heart rate variability") is finding ever wider application in assessing the risk of sudden cardiac arrest in patients who have already suffered a heart attack.

Doctors have always set great store by examining the pulse and have become highly proficient at it. In the third century BC Herophilus of Alexandria assessed separate phases of the pulse by using a clock of his own construction, which he took with him on visits to his patients. For centuries the pulse rate has been tested by all possible means, in the not unreasonable belief that it will provide a way to discover the secrets of how the heart and the entire body function. Only a few years ago medical students had to stand at the patient's bedside and define in a single breath such basic features of the pulse as its regularity, frequency, intensity, fullness, and tension. The terms used to encapsulate the main quality of a pulse must have seemed countless, as they spoke of a bigeminal pulse, a thready, or filiform, pulse, or when they ran out of adjectives, a paradoxical pulse. Surely in the present era of omnipotent technology all this knowledge has fallen by the wayside? Not at all—the 2000 edition of the renowned *Dorland's Medical Dictionary*, advertised as a compendium of the most essential information for medical practice in the third millennium, describes eighty-two different types of pulse!

Naturally, examining the pulse has had its stiffest competition from listening to the heart. The French doctor René Laënnec was the founder of auscultation; one day, to avoid placing his ear inappropriately close to the chest of a young female patient, he rolled a piece of paper into a tube, tied it with string and set it to her heart, never for a moment imagining that his invention would open up a whole new world of sounds—the ones that are literally closest to us, but that had been closed to our hearing until then. Arrhythmia provides the perfect example. A single extrasystole is like a slight stumble in a dance—one little sway that we don't even notice before we pick up the rhythm in the next step and it sweeps us onward. A heartbeat that is punctuated by recurring premature contractions makes us think that syncopation was not the original discovery of jazz musicians. In atrial fibrillation the pause between contractions changes, while the rhythmic accent shifts. The pace of a galloping horse can be heard in left heart failure (the "gallop rhythm"). The beating of a heart affected by a total block is interrupted at lengthy intervals by noisy "cannon fire" (when the atria and ventricles contract simultaneously), which is repeated by a faint echo of the atria contracting.

Echo was the name of a mountain nymph. The Greek myths give various explanations for how she came to personify a disembodied, recurring voice. After falling in unrequited love with Narcissus she sank into such despair that she began to disappear, until nothing was left of her but her voice. In another version, for keeping Zeus's love affairs secret Hera condemned Echo to repeat the last word of anyone who spoke to her. Not surprisingly, as new languages arose, they began to repeat her name. She found herself a home in them for ever, ultimately becoming one of the most frequently used words in modern medicine. Echo, echosonography, echocardiograph. . . . We penetrate the heart with sound waves, and they bounce back, returning to us as an echo, from which we can construct an image of the heart itself, one that is astoundingly precise in its details. The diagnostic equipment is developing so fast you might think it was trying to catch up with the perfect echolocation techniques of . . . bats.

By revealing the details of the anatomy of the heart or the power of its muscles to contract, the echocardiogram enables us to understand the causes of heartbeat disturbances. An electrocardiogram then enables us to diagnose them. An especially valuable tool is the around-the-clock ECG recorder, popularly named the Holter after an American doctor. It produces a diary, written by the heart, recording every single one of its contractions, and of course every, even the briefest, arrhythmia or ischemia. This record is an invaluable aid in everyday medical diagnostics. More refined analyses are also being developed to detect subtle asynchronicities in the action of the heart. Mathematicians and physicists are helping medical researchers with these extremely complex phenomena by applying the dynamics of nonlinear systems and chaos theory.

What a range of facilities there is nowadays for medical students trying to fathom the music of the heart! We lay a diaphragm fitted with an electronic amplifier over the sternum, at the point where the ribs join. It has six pairs of acoustic ducts coming out of it, just like the tube of an ordinary stethoscope. This allows six people to listen to the sounds issuing from the same point above the heart simultaneously. Meanwhile, the screen of a portable computer displays an electrocardiographic curve, and beneath it a phono-cardiogram—a nonstop recording of all the tones, murmurs, and other acoustic features produced by the heart. You can stop it, "freeze" it, and analyze it.

People have dreamed of freezing sounds, words, or even music since ancient times. Antiphanes, a member of Plato's household, told of a country where the winters were so harsh that words froze in the air. In summer, when they melted, the citizens found out what was talked about in winter, just as only in their old age did Plato's pupils begin to comprehend the meaning of the master's words that they had heard in their youth. Many centuries later, as described by Baldassare Castiglione, an Italian merchant made an expedition to the Ukraine for sable furs in winter. He got stuck on the frozen bank of the river Dnieper, from where he conducted negotiations with Muscovite merchants camping on the opposite bank. However, the words they shouted couldn't get across—they froze midway and hung in the air like icicles. So the Polish interpreters lit a fire in the middle of the river, but the thawed-out words contained such high prices that the Italian hurried back to his sunny country empty-handed.

But who could have outdone Baron Münchhausen in their tales of wintry lands?! In Gottfried August Bürger's version of his adventures, once while racing by sledge across the icy wastes of Russia, he told the postilion to play his horn the entire way. Not surprisingly, not a single sound came out of it—they all got stuck inside, frozen fast. That evening at the inn, where the horn was hung up by the fireplace, the music began to flow out of it, which was enough to make "cruelly frozen hearts melt with joy."

When a doctor "freezes" the heart on the operating table by lowering its temperature by a few degrees, he arrests its music and rhythm, because the heart stops beating. Mechanical pumps do its job for it, squeezing blood into the vessels. Once the operation is over, the heart is warmed up and goes back to work, emitting tones again. Driven by its rhythm, the blood starts circulating again.

When I was just starting out as a doctor, and Wrocław was in the grip of the worst winter of the century, at three in the morning a frozen man was brought in to us at the hospital. He had been found by the river Oder, where the temperature was down to minus 35°C. He was as stiff and cold as an icicle, he wasn't breathing, and his heart had stopped. The electrocardiogram showed a straight, horizontal line. The idea of reanimation had only just entered the debate, and we had no equipment at all. There were only two of us, myself and a nurse. I began to massage the heart, while she tried mouth-to-mouth resuscitation. With each breath the room was filled with the fumes of methylated spirits. The man's heart started functioning again after about an hour's massage, and the breathing shortly after. The next day the patient walked out on his own two feet, having earlier upbraided us for losing his packet of extra-strength cigarettes. Excitedly we sent a description of the incident to the *Lancet,* though we were unable to answer the editor's question about the temperature of the reanimated body. Almost thirty years later, the same periodical featured an article about an accident that happened to a Norwegian lady skiing champion, who fell into a deep crevasse in the far north of her country. She was brought out of it two hours later in a lifeless state, with a body temperature of 13.7°C, and was taken by rescue plane to Tromsø. Her heart got going again only after several hours of pumping her blood through an extracorporeal blood-warming device. She left the hospital after five months of rehabilitation. Similar cases have lately prompted the idea of fitting intensive care units, where patients resuscitated out of doors are taken, with mattresses that cool the body by at least a few degrees, in the hope of delaying the moment when irreversible brain damage occurs and restoring the pulse and heartbeat more quickly and easily.

Several thousand Americans cannot have their pulse taken or their blood pressure tested, though some of them move about fairly easily. They have small pumps sewn into the heart that help the blood to flow from the left chamber into the aorta continuously, without pulsating. There are also some patients alive in this world whose heart has been removed and replaced with an artificial one, the size of a grapefruit, entirely made of plastic and titanium, described by the experts as an expression of the most advanced technology man has ever carried inside himself. Electrical pacemakers are also in common use, and the range of drugs to prevent arrhythmia is extremely wide and still growing. Yet in some cases the strongest drugs can prove disappointing, while a simple word can help.

Years ago Jerzy Turowicz, editor in chief of Poland's leading Catholic weekly, *Tygodnik Powszechny,* was admitted to our hospital with a serious generalized infection. We managed to get it under control, but there was still some arrhythmia. His heart was beating at a bad, ominous rhythm, of a kind that doesn't simply recede by itself, but presages the worst possible danger. We applied some strong drugs—to no effect. We had reached the limits of our powers. One evening I went to see Jerzy in his private room, listened to his heart and went home, feeling depressed by my own helplessness. Early the next morning I put my stethoscope to his heart again and heard a pure, steady, regular heart beat. I couldn't believe my own ears, but the ECG recording brought confirmation. In amazement I asked him: "Did something happen last night, Jerzy?" Smiling in his usual gentle, kindly way he said: "Actually, His Holiness the Pope called me after midnight from the Vatican."

The mystery of how blood circulates within the human body was discovered almost two hundred years after the discovery that the earth and the planets revolve around the sun. Our lengthy inability to recognize something so vital, relevant to every single one of us, seems almost incomprehensible, especially as the set of experiments needed to establish this truth could have been devised and performed without any obstacles for several thousand years. William Harvey, who discovered the secret of blood circulation, was an experienced anatomist and pathologist and a scholar of insatiable curiosity. Before working on man, he performed dissections of about two hundred different animals, including an ostrich, which in early-seventeenth-century London was not exactly the simplest of matters. Then, with the help of some simple incisions and by bandaging the human hand, he confirmed that blood flows away from the heart along the arteries and back toward it along the veins.

Comparing the orbit of the planets around the sun and the circulation of blood within the human body makes us think of music. A tradition derived from Pythagoras and Plato compared the cosmos to a musical instrument, creating harmony out of discordant elements. It was the rhythmic motion of the planets that was the source of music. The music of the celestial spheres, the expression of perfect harmony, is always resonating around us, although we can never hear it, just as we cannot hear the rhythmic hum of our blood, as it is with us from birth. It reaches us only in rare moments when the body's harmony is deeply disturbed, when it is ill, in sickness.

My beloved *Oxford Companion to Music* defines rhythm as the countenance of music, turned to face time. How might we relate that to the rhythm of the heart?

A surge of blood flows to billions of our cells, and, like an ocean wave that licks at the sandy shore, it laps against them before flowing away again, to return after a fixed interval. Our large internal organs, and the cells they are made of, are endlessly rocked by waves that ebb and flow. They can feel and hear the roar and rhythm of the blood, which "binds together distant shores / with a thread of mutual agreement" and tells them about the flow of time.

VII. A PURIFYING POWER

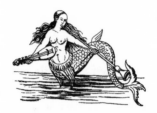

Six hundred years ago Petrarch claimed that if you were to take a thousand people suffering from a given illness, hand half of them over to a doctor, and leave the other half to themselves, the ones left on their own would have a better chance of recovery. Over the centuries it has often been said that the difference between a good doctor and a bad one is vast, but there isn't any difference between a good doctor and no doctor. Harvard biochemist Lawrence J. Henderson reckoned that only from about 1910, for the first time ever, did the average patient who consulted a doctor chosen at random have a more than 50% chance of benefiting from the visit. If that was the case, how could medicine have functioned for so many thousands of years? How do we explain all the recoveries? Surely the doctors had something to do with them, all but the most second-rate practitioners, perhaps?

Hippocrates' explanation for this paradox was the healing power of nature. In nature itself, he taught, beneficent, therapeutic powers and a healing force (the *vis medicatrix naturae*) lie dormant. One should trust in nature, keeping a close watch at a patient's bedside to see how it acts; one should help it, and never do harm. That too was the original meaning of the aphorism, repeated as often nowadays as centuries ago—*primum non nocere:* above all, do no harm. The doctor is meant to be nature's helper, not its teacher: he should be the *minister,* not the *magister naturae.* The followers of Hippocrates saw how the crisis of an illness was accompanied by sweating, diarrhea, vomiting, suppuration, catarrh, coughing up phlegm, and bleeding. They interpreted these symptoms as proof that the body contains natural powers to restore the balance of the humors that determine health, to rid itself of bad juices and harmful elements—to purify itself. And as early as pre-Hippocratic Greece the forerunners of doctors were known as "purifiers" (*kathartai*), and were mentioned in the same breath as the magi, who knew love charms and sold amulets and talismans to magic away illness. People believed that the gods sent down disease as a punishment, so the task of the doctor-chiromancer was to identify and demonstrate how to purify oneself from sin, in order to return to health. Thus, in *The Iliad,* when plague breaks out among the Greek troops, Kalchas, augur for the Achaians, describes the ways of making purifying sacrifices.

Every single entry into the temple of Asclepius was preceded by fasting, ablutions, and sacrifices. The culmination of these rituals, the dramatic nocturnal events in the temple that restored health, contained an element of the stage, the hallmarks of theater—it was like a play, a work of art. The word *katharsis* also connected it with art.

The concept of *katharsis* is usually traced back to Pythagoras, but the term appeared much earlier, at the beginning of Greek art—in the chorus (the *khoreia*), which was a combination of music and dance, poetry and song. Performed during mysteries and rites, the chorus served to soothe and calm the emotions, and "in contemporary language, to purify the soul," that is, to perform *katharsis.* In the third century BC, Pseudo-Plutarch, author of a famous treatise, *De Musica,* pointed out that it shared its origins with medicine. He wrote: "Homer . . . created the character of Achilles, who soothed the anger he felt toward Agamemnon with music, which he had learned from the extremely wise Chiron." Thus, *katharsis* could have been the gift of Chiron, the centaur who brought up and educated Asclepius, "Chiron, the teacher of music, justice, and medicine all in one."

The Pythagoreans believed that the soul was imprisoned in the body as a punishment for its faults and would be freed once purified of them. They regarded this purification as man's loftiest aim and adopted the idea that it was possible thanks to music. According to the neo-Platonic philosopher Iamblichus: "The Pythagoreans . . . cleansed the body by means of medicine, and the soul by means of music." Thus, they believed, for example, that when intoxicated by Bacchic music, the soul was liberated and temporarily left the body. For the same reason they regarded music as an exceptional state, a special gift of the gods.

However, Aristotle was the first to make *katharsis* the mysterious enigma that it remains to this day. In his *Politics* he brings up the word *katharsis* and promises to discuss it in detail later on, in view of its key significance. However, he returns to it only once more, in his *Poetics,* where he addresses the issue tersely and ambiguously. By doing this he opened the way for the innumerable interpretations that have accumulated over the centuries. Some people have assumed that the text about *katharsis* in the *Poetics* has been "amputated by an unknown censor"; others have expressed the view that it was the subject of a separate, irretrievably lost essay. Some have even said in hushed tones that the Stagirite deliberately left the crucial issue of art open ended, because it eludes unambiguous interpretation. Did he perhaps notice that in the first syllable of the word he meant to define an ancient, unfathomed mystery lay spellbound? We first find "Ka" at the beginning of the history of ancient Egypt as "one of the most difficult concepts for the Western mind to grasp." It was associated with the force that sustains life, the power of creation, and the soul of man. Centuries earlier, at the dawn of Hindu civilization, Ka was the name of the father of the gods, the life-giving element that pervaded the world. The god's name Ka meant "Who?"—and the first reaction to it was "boundless awe."

The brevity of Aristotle's remark and the age-old debates that it prompted remind us of another episode that has its roots in ancient Greece—the story of Fermat's great theorem. Pierre de Fermat, a seventeenth-century lawyer from Toulouse, made significant discoveries in the theory of numbers and achieved fame in his own lifetime. He spent all his spare time reading the works of the ancient mathematicians. When he died, he was found with a copy of *Arithmetic,* by the Greek mathematician Diophantus, who lived in the third century BC. On reading about a problem to do with the division of a square into the sum of two other squares, Fermat made a brilliant generalization, encapsulated it in a theorem, and wrote in the margin: "It is impossible for any number which is a power greater than the second to be written as a sum of two powers. I have a truly marvelous demonstration of this proposition that this margin is too narrow to contain." Fermat's proof has never been found. The comment written in the margin drove the level-headed René Descartes to despair, and for generations of mathematicians it has been an endless incentive for research. What is known as Fermat's great, or last, theorem is acknowledged as the most famous mathematical problem of all time, not because of its importance to algebra, but as a symbol of something that defies the human mind, something unattainable and impossible. European academies have offered large rewards for proof of the theorem, and thousands of mathematicians and keen enthusiasts have thought they have found it, but the only things they ever really found were errors in their own reasoning. Thanks to this research, which went on for three hundred years, some new branches of mathematics were developed. Finally, in 1995 British mathematician Andrew Wiles presented the unshakable proof that settled the matter. "Fermat's last theorem was a theorem at last."

Katharsis has not yet encountered its own Andrew Wiles. But does it really need one? What did the phenomenal Briton actually present in his proof, which "it is doubtful if more than a few dozen mathematicians in the entire world are in a position to fully understand"? Wiles proved that a certain equation cannot have defined, unambiguous solutions. (To be more precise, he showed that "the equation $z^n = x^n + y^n$ has no whole-number solutions for any power greater than 2." In simple terms that is the essence of Fermat's last theorem.) Do we need mathematical proof that there is no unambiguous solution to *katharsis*? Was that perhaps why Aristotle put the issue as he did and not otherwise? Let's hear how he defined *katharsis* in his *Poetics* when writing about tragedy, which he regarded as the highest form of art. His famous definition goes as follows: "Tragedy is an imitation of an action that is serious, complete, and of a certain magnitude; in language embellished with each kind of artistic ornament, the several kinds being found in separate parts of the play; in the form of action, not of narrative; through pity and fear effecting the proper purgation of these emotions."

Aristotle's words have stirred endless debate over whether he meant purification of the emotions, or purifying the mind from emotions. "In other words, the sublimation, or the discharge of emotions? Improving them, or getting free of them?" Was he talking about perfecting and idealizing our emotions, or ridding ourselves of an excess of disturbing, destructive emotions, in order to achieve inner peace? For a long time people tended toward the first interpretation, but nowadays the second generally takes precedence.

There is also contention over whether Aristotle sourced *katharsis* from medicine (*katharsis peri to soma*, corresponding to the Latin *purgatio*), or from religious cult (*katharsis peri to psyche*, the Latin *purificatio*). The medical sources were undoubtedly closer to him, and in mentioning *katharsis* in his *Politics* with reference to music, he used medical terminology (*iatreia kai katharsis*) in its technical sense, just as Hippocrates and his pupils used it. Thus, *katharsis* contains both a medical and an Orphic element. The Orphic element is the magical effect of music, which is capable of altering the ordinary course of events, subverting natural laws, restoring man to health, and elevating him to the godhead, but also of hurling him into the abyss of evil. Aristotle recalled that when Orpheus played and sang, people and animals stood entranced, rivers changed their course, trees tore their roots from the earth and stepped toward him, and even boulders rolled to his feet. By associating *katharsis* with *mimesis,* Aristotle "understood the purification of the emotions to be a natural psychological and biological process."

To explain the powerful effect of art, the Pythagoreans accepted the idea of a kinship between movement and sound and the soul. On the one hand, dance movements or musical sounds express emotions, and on the other, they evoke them, by having an effect on the soul. "Sounds find a resonance in the soul and harmonize with it. It is like with two lyres: when we strike one, the other one that's near it responds."

Music restored health through purification of the soul. Aristotle wrote that some people, under the influence of a melody that puts their soul in a state of rapture, feel soothed, as if they had taken medicine or a calming remedy. There were attempts to pacify lunatics with music, on the other hand, by impressing "upon their disorganised souls the magically numerical and cosmic order, attuning them, as it were, to the proportions of the universe." Treating illnesses of the body far more rarely gets a men-

tion, but it is worth remembering that paeans were originally incantations against disease and death.

Although barely a dozen ancient Greek tunes have survived, some
of them only in extracts, interest in Greek music is arguably
greater than in that of any other period in the history of ancient
music. "Do not bid me live without music," sings the choir of old
men in Euripides, and this cry is echoed in a poem by Polish poet
Józef Czechowicz (1903–1939): "Protect us from an empty life
without music and song." The expressions "without music,"
"without the choir," "without a lyre" were commonly associated
with the cruelties of war, with the vengeance of the Furies, and
with death. Images of happiness in Greek poetry resonate with
music, and their festivities were full of dancing, singing, and lyre
or aulos playing. Music strengthened or weakened the character,
created order or anarchy, brought peace or unrest. In the ninth
century BC the musician Thaletas was appointed to help Lycur-
gus, the Spartan lawgiver. Once during a civil war the Delphic oracle advised summoning the composer Terpander, who could
calm the city with music. Plato counseled the guardians of his
ideal state to base the principles of the republic on music.

Pythagoras's dazzling discovery that musical consonances, or
intervals, are reflected in simple numerical ratios was the starting
point for the theory of beauty based on order and proportion. The
Greeks expressed the emotional power of a melody and its effect
on the soul within the science of "the ethos of music." They said
that the soul could be put into a good or bad *ethos* (character). The
Pythagoreans placed special emphasis on distinguishing good music from bad, in order "in a matter as morally and socially important as music not to admit freedom and the associated risks." The
science of the ethos was one of the most original of the Greeks'
aesthetic theories, which exerted a direct influence on medicine.

In their view, the educational and spiritual effect of music depended above all on the musical mode (or modal scale), which we

might roughly define as corresponding to our musical key. Each Greek tribe used a different mode. There were extreme contrasts between the Dorian and the Phrygian modes. The former apparently sounded austere, deep, and low and was played on the lyre and the kithara, while the latter sounded high, shrill, and passionate and was played on pipes as part of the cult of Dionysus. The Greeks regarded their old music, the Dorian, as a source of strength and calm, while the Phrygian—a later invasion from Asia—was exciting and orgiastic. Plato ascribed a positive ethos to the former and a negative ethos to the latter. In his *Metaphysics* Aristotle wrote that the Dorian mode produces "a moderate and settled temper," while the Phrygian mode evokes "enthusiasm." Between these extremes there were various intermediate modes, including the Aeolian and the Ionian, among others. What exactly gave these modes such emotional force? "What made Dorian virile and bellicose; Hypodorian, majestic and stable; Mixolydian, pathetic and plaintive; Phrygian, agitated and Bacchic; Hypophrygian, active; Lydian, mournful; Hypolydian, dissolute and voluptuous?" Why in *The Republic* does Socrates say that "the Mixolydian and the hyper-Lydian modes are dirgelike and ought to be done away with, for they are useless 'even to women'"? We do not know, and there is nothing to imply that we ever will. "No one individual trait creates an ethos: neither the modal structure, nor the pitch, nor the bifocal nature of some tunes." Some people cherish the hope that knowledge of the *maqam* system—the Islamic music of the Orient, which also relies on modal scales, and to which therapeutic qualities are ascribed—will help them to understand ethos. The systematized, formal structures of Islamic melodies were supposed to cure not only the emotions but also physical complaints: Rast healed the eyes, Iraq got rid of heart palpitations, and Isfahan cured colds.

Never since has the connection between music and therapy been as direct as in ancient Greece. However, musicians have on occasion found themselves playing the role of doctors. When Count Keyserling "was suffering from the bane of insomnia, for which there is no consolation," he placed an order with Johann Sebastian Bach for . . . soporific music. Apparently Bach was reluctant to take on this incongruous commission, though it was fortified with the condition that the composition be light and charming. A pleasant aria came into being, with thirty variations full of virtuoso brilliance, known as the Goldberg Variations after Bach's favorite pupil, who spent night after night playing them to the count on the harpsichord. There is no doubting that the curative effect was excellent, because the master gained a regular stipend from the count, and his pupil was given "a golden vessel filled with louis d'or."

Modern research by American pediatricians based on sensitive recordings of the functions of the brain indicates that four-month-old babies prefer consonances to dissonances. Consonances are the intervals that sound pleasant to the ear, built upon the simple, Pythagorean proportions of natural numbers, such as an octave (1:2), a fifth (2:3), or a fourth (3:4). Their countertype are dissonances, such as a minor second. If we may draw conclusions from the behavior of four-month-old babies, in the brain of a sick person music based on consonances does not arouse the same centers as a string of dissonances. It tunes the brain like an instrument, putting it in a pure, good, and positive mood. Doesn't that sound similar to the ancient Greek science concerning the ethos of music?!

Regardless of whether or not small babies prefer consonances to dissonances as a result of having heard music while still in their mother's womb, the human brain comes into the world with a natural ability to be perceptive and to extract certain musical regularities from the surrounding world. The high incidence of octaves and fifths in the music of cultures that are very far apart might be a consequence of the structure of our auditory organs.

Every one of us has a tiny harp inside his ear. The basilar membrane of the cochlea in the inner ear is made of flexible, transverse fibers, shorter at the base, and many times longer at the top of the cochlea. This set of fibers looks like the strings of a harp or a piano. The world's sounds enter the ear via the auditory canal and go on past the tympanic membrane (eardrum) and tiny ossicles until they reach the cochlea. They plunge into the fluid that fills it and reach the basilar membrane in a wave. The length of this incoming wave, that is, the pitch of the sound, determines which fibers in the cochlea's basilar membrane, the ear's harp, will start to ripple and vibrate. Signals from the vibrating fibers are collected by special sensory cells, called hair cells, which then send them along nerves to the brain. The distances between the hair cells in the cochlea's membrane correspond to steps on the chromatic scale. The basis for their arrangement are the sets of harmonic tones that are a component of each sound. The composer Leonard Bernstein called harmonic tones "the built-in preordained universal" and "common origin" of all music. Might this universe be built into us too?

It is hard to imagine that these questions bothered Neanderthal man, yet the excavated pipes that he used to play fifty thousand years ago, made of bear or deer bones, can produce "many different types of scales . . . and the sounds are pure and haunting." Based on comparisons of the singing of birds, whales, and humans, some researchers suspect the existence of a single, Platonic world of music that is still waiting to be discovered. The state of Georgia in the U.S.A. has decided not to wait any longer for the results of this highly interesting but complex research and has taken action. Since 1999 the christening of every young citizen of Georgia takes place to the accompaniment of music by Mozart. The state's lawmakers must have been pleased when they read the observations of some American neonatologists that were published a year later. From them it appears that among premature babies being treated in intensive care units, music has a favorable effect on their mood, perception of pain, heart rate, blood pressure, weight gain, and even the saturation of their blood with oxygen! So was Novalis right two hundred years ago when he wrote: "Every disease is a musical problem, every cure a musical solution"?

VIII. SUFFERING

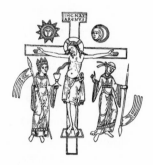

It is hard to imagine a more magnificent start to the new millennium—in its very first weeks the entire human genetic code was deciphered and published, nucleotide after nucleotide, three billion letters. Medicine became molecular and entered the new, "postgenomic" era. As if not overly concerned that the considerable majority of the genome remains incomprehensible to us, it is already publicizing its latest field, known as proteomics, which aims to recognize every single nuance of the structure and function of proteins, a task many times more complex than interpreting the human genome. More and more people are convinced that the truly staggering achievements are still ahead of us. The problem of correcting distorted genetic codes is still outstanding but is bound to be solved at some point. This is one of the optimistic scenarios for medicine in the near future—we are ousting illness and suffering from our consciousness.

As soon as we enter hospital wards and corridors, we gain some dramatic insight into the weakness and frailty of human nature.

Here the mystery of physical pain is most forcefully revealed, which in the words of John Paul II "poses to the human mind one of the most poignant questions." Here we may find endless human suffering and loneliness. But it is also a place of hope—the hopes of the patients, who feel the will to live, and the hopes of their friends and relatives who share their confidence that they'll soon show an improvement heralding a return to health. Naturally, doctors, nurses, and the entire hospital staff play their part in the recovery of these hopes. They strive to restore ties with the rest of the healthy world that have been damaged, or sometimes completely broken by illness. If in doing this they manage to bring together competence and talent, perseverance and goodwill, they are on the ideal path toward building a partnership between sick people and those who come to relieve their suffering, free them from illness and return them to health. A clinic or a hospital department can represent this sort of partnership.

In the eyes of the world pain and suffering are a terrible thing, futile and destructive, especially when children have to suffer, or when innocent people meet with an accident, become disabled, or contract a fatal illness. "Who committed the sin that caused him to be born blind?" the disciples asked Christ. "He or his parents?" "Neither—it was no sin on this man's part, nor on his parents' part. Rather, it was to let God's work be revealed in him." So it's a test sent down to us by God? An improving test of suffering that allows the strength of the spirit to be revealed when the flesh is weak? Nowadays this idea has been called into question. The modern cult of success requires us to be eternally young and healthy. The world of mass culture does not accept pain or suffering—it finds them repulsive. Following the launch of stress-free education we have set about achieving the full "exorcism of pain from the world."

This is not a new idea, although never before has it been conceived on such a large scale. From the dawn of time magicians and

shamans—the forerunners of doctors—tried to alleviate pain.
They knew and applied plant extracts, from which thousands of
years later the two major groups of analgesic drugs were developed: salicylates and opiates.

No drugs have been a more faithful companion to man throughout his history than salicylates, the forebears of aspirin. Almost
four thousand years ago the Ebers Papyrus advised coating the
small of the back and the stomach with an extract of myrtle leaves
to get rid of rheumatic pains. Hippocrates applied infusions of
poplar in eye diseases, and sap from willow bark to treat fever and
labor pains. These plants and trees are abundant in compounds
derived from salicylic acid, which gets its name from them (in
Latin, *salix* is a willow tree). For thousands of years they have
helped to relieve pain, bring down fever, and reduce inflammation. Their healing properties were known to the Chinese, the
Amerindians, and the Hottentots of southern Africa. The British
are proud of the fact that the first "clinical research" was conducted in the mid-eighteenth century by an Oxfordshire parish
priest, the Reverend Edward Stone. By chance he happened to
taste some willow bark and found it surprisingly bitter, a flavor
that reminded him of an extract from the bark of the quinine tree,
which was used to treat malaria. The Reverend Stone was a fol-
lower of the doctrine of signatures and believed that in the place
where an illness spreads the remedy to cure it must also be found.
As "willow delights in a moist and wet soil, where ague chiefly
abounds," he gathered a pound of willow bark, dried it for three
months in a baking oven, and applied it to fifty people suffering
from rheumatism. The results confirmed that his theory was
right. They were excellent, as he reported in a special letter to the
Royal Society. Throughout the next century work continued to
refine salicylates from plant products and to synthesize them
chemically. In 1899 the laboratories of pharmaceutical firm Bayer
brought a simple, synthetic derivative of salicylic acid onto the

market—aspirin. It has since become the most popular drug in the world, partly because of its anticoagulant properties that prevent heart attacks, which were only discovered and documented in the past few decades. The phenomenal success of aspirin has stimulated the production of many drugs that act in a similar way.

The intoxicating and analgesic effect of opium, obtained from poppy sap, was already known to the Sumerians, but it was the Greek empiricists who introduced it into therapy in the third century BC. "Non interesse quod morbum faciat, sed quid tollat" (It is not important what an illness causes, but what cures it), said Celsus at the dawn of the Christian era, chiming in with the pragmatic empiricists. In these words we can hear a portent of palliative medicine, which developed at the same time, with opiates as its main weapon.

The inability to control pain, apart from infections that could be contracted during an operation, was the main obstacle to the development of surgery. In the late eighteenth century nitrous oxide was synthesized, otherwise known as laughing gas. It even gained popularity in the London circles of revelers, who livened up their entertainments with stupefacients, but the idea of applying it in surgery was unheard of. In those days mesmerism was widespread, a practice that relied on elements of suggestion or hypnosis, based on a belief in cosmic forces known as "animal magnetism." Arousing them in the patient's body was supposed to reestablish contact with the universe, relieve pain, and remove illness. As Franz Anton Mesmer wrote: "A fluid that pervades the entire universe in waves that resemble the ebb and flow of the tide links together all the heavenly bodies, which in this way exert an influence on all parts of living beings and can strengthen or weaken the properties of matter and organic bodies, such as their weight, cohesion, electricity, etc. This fluid . . . cures all illnesses immediately . . . ; it is what makes drugs, crises and any treatment effective." The magnetic influence of the universe and of people on themselves had many supporters in the age of romanticism and had a significant effect on surgery. The breakthrough came in the 1840s, first arriving from the New World.

We owe general anesthetics to two American dentists. Horace Wells tested nitrous oxide first on himself before undergoing a tooth extraction, and then on several of his patients. Next he decided to make a public demonstration before an audience of medical students at a lecture hall in Boston. When the anesthetized patient cried out, Wells was mocked and booed by the audience. He lost heart, but his lack of success encouraged another dentist to conduct some tests using ether. Just over a year later the first painless surgical operation was performed in Boston before a medical audience. The sensational news raced around the world. In the years that followed chloroform began to take the place of ether. Those who opposed narcosis had to think again when the royal doctor anesthetized Queen Victoria during childbirth, and the delivery was a success.

We only have to look at old prints showing operations performed without anesthetic, such as sawing off a leg, to realize what the introduction of narcosis meant. However, pain does not only set in physically. Obsessive thoughts going round and round in circles can be no less a torture than the rack, as a fevered mind spins around one central point, like a maddened carousel that we cannot stop, despite feeling worse with every turn. The first mechanical device to inflict mental possession was invented by Aphrodite to help Jason gain the favor of the sorceress Medea, without which he would never obtain the Golden Fleece. She took a wryneck, a bird that twists its neck with a sudden jerking movement, and "fixed it with bonds that could not be untied to a little wheel with four spokes. Now the circular motion of the wheel would forever accompany the jerky twisting of the bird's neck." Thus, she made a mechanism that "imposes an obsessive circular motion on the mind, uproots it from its inertia," and makes it go round and round incessantly. From then on Medea's mind was driven by dreams of Jason; she used all her magic powers to rescue the foreigner, at the cost of destroying her own family. No one was more predestined than Aphrodite to invent the possession machine, "for erotic possession is the starting point for any possession."

There are events that "break so vast a Heart," putting it in a state of paralysis, and causing a pain that only time can change into numbness.

> After great pain, a formal feeling comes—
> The Nerves sit ceremonious, like Tombs—
> The stiff Heart questions 'was it He, that bore,'
> And 'Yesterday, or Centuries before?'
>
> The Feet, mechanical, go round—
> A Wooden way
> Of Ground, or Air, or Ought—
> Regardless grown,
> A Quartz contentment, like a stone—

Sometimes psychological shock is so intense that it causes profound lethargy. This deathlike state, which no one knew how to distinguish from real death, was particularly feared in the eighteenth and nineteenth centuries. Yet people suffering from phantom pain, following the amputation of a leg, for example, have said that they would prefer death to the suffering they endure, for which medicine has a hard time finding a remedy—a ghost pain, a phantom still occupying the space where a part that has gone for ever used to be.

If only we knew how to resist pain as well as the Roman Stoic philosopher Epictetus did! When he was still a slave, he had to bear his master's cruelties without a word of complaint. He treated his own body as a form of clothing. He resembled Socrates in saying that a philosopher should be indifferent to physical ailments and public applause. Where should we seek help in suffering? The loving presence of our nearest and dearest, their words of comfort and good cheer are the "spiritual medicine" that restores our will to live and to fight for life. "To comfort someone means to raise his suffering to the height of dignity in his own eyes." Turning suffering into a metaphor makes the pain easier to bear. That's how it works when we tell ourselves we're suffering for someone or something else. Sometimes it helps a great deal. "If I'm suffering now, then—like in communicating vessels—it reduces someone else's suffering," wrote Polish novelist Stefan Chwin in an essay on the nature of pain. It's worth reminding the patient that we are always something more than the one single meaning the surrounding world tries to impose on us, the world of simplified generalizations and reductions, the world of clumsy divisions. In short, we have to make sense of pain; only then can we bear it and not be condemned to barren torment.

Putting up resistance to suffering and refusing to accept it have caused us to call God into question since time immemorial. After all, suffering is hard to understand—even those who believe in God find it inexplicable, especially the fact that having faith doesn't mean an end to suffering. Let's hear the view of John Paul II, who always tried to be there for those who suffer and who had already given suffering thorough consideration long before it started to weigh down very heavily upon him too. He confirms its presence by writing: "Humanity undergoes a Calvary of suffering." And in the following words he tells us: "Could God have justified Himself before human history, so full of suffering, without placing Christ's Cross at the center of that history? . . . The crucified Christ is proof of God's solidarity with man in suffering.

God places Himself on the side of man. He does so in a radical way." We also hear his fine words about the "Heavenly Doctor," to whom we turn, because he "possesses the power to heal our numerous weaknesses, very varied, but always real and demanding immediate help, from physical illnesses to the moral ailments that are sins."

In a hospital at night, a long scream of pain pierces the silence. Until recently this was a common scenario, but nowadays the screams have been silenced and suffering has lost its voice. The range of analgesic drugs has become very wide, and there are just as many ways of administering them around the clock, so we stop pain in its tracks and wipe it out of our minds. But even though it's quieter—soundless, in fact—suffering hasn't actually gone away for good. There are times when it crosses the limit, and when it does, it wreaks havoc. It kills the patient's sense of closeness and sympathy. The bond is broken, and there's a lack of response, just as if the person suffering were locked in another world. The burden falling on the doctor and nurses increases sharply. Words become insufficient, inadequate. The doctor's hand shrinks from the door handle when there's a patient lying on the other side whom he has no more to offer. But there is still one thing left: his presence, the result of plain human solidarity. Being there is the doctor's ultimate duty.

You can put a stop to endless suffering by taking life. The euthanasia debate covers a broad range of opinion. The voice of medicine shouldn't be the only one entitled to settle the argument, but the medical world has a duty to take a stance on it.

The fact that both patient and doctor share a sense of hopelessness when suffering refuses to subside despite full palliative treatment does not justify euthanasia, because it violates the essential situation of medicine: the relationship between patient and doctor. It is inevitably bound to introduce a mistrust and fear of doctors and nurses into society. A patient's apparently voluntary agreement to undergo euthanasia could be the result of depression or, even worse, the upshot of pressure from his family acting out of their own selfish motives. Ultimately it is the duty of society, and especially the medical world, to protect its weakest members—the sick, old, disabled, poor, ethnic minorities, and so on. In an extreme scenario these people could be rejected by society, or even see themselves as unproductive and a burden on others—and on that basis be regarded as candidates for euthanasia.

In performing euthanasia the doctor himself commits the act of taking life, by injecting poison, for example. A subtler method which has a growing number of supporters is medically assisted suicide, when a doctor helps the patient to take his own life, for example, by taking an overdose of a drug that was designed only to relieve pain. Thus, some people say that assisted suicide is merely one of today's varieties of suicide.

Suicide is shocking. It disturbs the deepest layers of our soul much more acutely than natural death, and it always prompts the same empty, crushing questions: was there no way it could have been avoided? Couldn't I have done something to save that life? This reaction contains sympathy and solidarity with human fate, as well as terror at the sight of the self-preservation instinct breaking down. It also expresses our inability to understand and accept suffering, because suicide is born of suffering, spiritual and physical. Driven to extreme measures when he lost in love, Werther could no longer go on living. The moment misery exhausts our given supply of strength to live, as soon as an individual crosses the limit of suffering that he can bear, as Goethe says in Werther's words, suicide becomes a natural act. Macbeth too finds no salvation in the doctor as he despairingly calls for help for his murdering wife:

> Cure her of that.
> Canst thou not minister to a mind diseas'd,
> Pluck from the memory a rooted sorrow,

Raze out the written troubles of the brain,
And with some sweet oblivious antidote
Cleanse the stuff'd bosom of that perilous stuff
Which weighs upon the heart?

Not an easy task to come up to. The doctor witnesses pain and suffering on a daily basis, things the world regards as terrible, futile, and destructive. He stands before "reality with a thousand faces," before "a riddle we cannot solve to our satisfaction, in a purely human way." He sees how the idea of suicide is born in physical suffering. It has been with us since the dawn of history; it was debated by the ancient Greeks, was approved in extreme situations by Marcus Aurelius and Seneca, was ardently censured and at the same time defended by Jean-Jacques Rousseau in *The New Heloise,* and is still discussed by modern thinkers, including the Romanian writer Emile Cioran (1911–1995), who said that "what makes life bearable is the thought that one can leave it."

But should the doctor set his hand to suicide? Is it a question of ethics, morality, or law? Opinion is divided, from the extreme view that the doctor is "a paid accomplice in dealing death" to the complete opposite, which sees him as "the final depository of human dignity." These sentiments take on particular topicality when the law encroaches on the delicate issue of ethics and—as happened recently in Holland and Belgium—sanctions euthanasia and medically assisted suicide. Holland and Belgium remain isolated examples. In other countries the medical societies as well as the legal regulations have rejected this attitude. To those who are uncertain or misguided, subjected to a widening wave of relativism, let us say loud and clear: it is not allowed—Polish law forbids it, and the penal code punishes doctors who assist in suicides.

I'd like to finish with a personal observation. Those in favour of euthanasia and assisted suicide base their opinion on the convic-

tion that the doctor's diagnosis is indisputably correct. Dear
reader, if you only knew how often I've been wrong in my medical
prognosis! How many times a year it happens! If death depended
on my medical judgment (unanimously supported by a number of
my expert colleagues), how many fewer people would be walking
the earth today!

IX. EXITUS

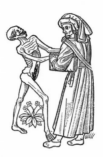

The jolting line of the temperature graph breaks off. The pulse and blood pressure recording fades out. The ECG shows a flat horizontal line. "Like a string when the concert's over," as Zbigniew Herbert put it. Right across the temperature chart, in one sweep of the pen, the word *Exitus* is written. Time. Signature. Doctor's stamp.

And before that?

> I've seen a Dying Eye
> Run round and round a Room—
> In search of Something—as it seemed
> Then Cloudier become—
> And then—obscure with Fog—
> And then—be soldered down
> Without disclosing what it be
> 'Twere blessed to have seen—

Is it then, at the final moment, that extraordinary clarity of vision comes over us? A sort of extra element of mystery at the moment of revelation? Does the hitherto hidden countenance of the world suddenly reveal itself? And can we take it in, understand it, and finally give it a name?

> Is it only then, when to eyes wide open in final surprise
> night will start falling on giant wing,
> Is it then you'll let hands going cold, shuddering like shades on
> the counterpane,
> strike out your real name?

The doctor can hear the footsteps of death approaching in a patient's heart and can see its shadow on his face. He recognizes the moment when it takes the patient into its possession. Hippocrates looked for portents of the irreversible end and left the following description of them for his pupils: "In a severe fever or brain disease keep this in mind . . : When the patient drags his hands across his face, tries to grasp at something in midair, picks crumbs or strands from his clothing, or tiny specks off the wall, it is all an unmistakable omen." Many years later some eminent French doctors must have seen patients making the same small, rapid, raking movement with their fingers and said: *Ils font ses petits paquets*—that is, "They're packing up for the journey." A person who sinks into a hepatic coma, however, lets us know when he is past the point of no return by stretching out his arms and waving at us. "He's waving good-bye," as some doctors put it. As if he were on a train leaving the station, waving out of the window at us, standing on the platform to bid him farewell.

For Talleyrand advance knowledge of the date of his death would determine the result of the final great game he initiated. He sought the advice of at least five doctors. However, he may have been relying more on his close acquaintance with Time. After all, he had survived the *ancien régime,* the Revolution, Napoleon, the Treaty of Vienna, and the Restoration—and in every single one of these episodes he had pulled the strings of history, steering the politics of France and Europe. "The supreme diplomat of the century," as Goethe said of him. He used his incisive intelligence to serve ever-changing regimes and systems. For all that, he became the object of universal contempt, which "would have got under his skin if he hadn't kept it on the outside, in the faintly twisted corners of his lips." Napoleon, whose minister he was, flew at him with fists flying, shouting: "You are a shit in silk stockings, Sir!" The Duchess d'Abrantès put it more subtly, saying: "Our dear friend, the eternal traitor Talleyrand—the only man who has succeeded in betraying everyone and everything, with the exception of style."

Talleyrand—a man of inscrutable countenance, impeccable manners, the master of ceremonies—told the doctor from whom he wanted to elicit the date of his death: "There's nothing I fear so much as improper protocol." At the time he was reading François Fénelon's work on the futility and transience of all the kingdoms of this world, except for the eternal kingdom of God's children. He wrote in the margin, "Beautiful!" and decided that his place was in that very kingdom. However, it seemed completely unattainable. He could not even count on a church funeral, for at least two reasons. During the Revolution he had ordained some lay bishops, on top of which, though himself a bishop of the Catholic Church, he had broken his vows and married.

So then he prepared his final game, as ever right down to the last detail and in total secrecy. Four months before he died, he met with the cardinal of Paris. The church was expecting him to make a public confession of the entire list of his sins; by doing so he would strike out his entire life. This was when he displayed his political genius to the full once more. Talleyrand knew that in politics what is more important than the text of a document is the time when you sign it. Throughout his life he was a past master at dragging out decisions. As his health declined more and more each day and he could no longer leave his bed, he refused to place his signature on four successive versions of his confession of repentance, as presented to him by the church. Finally he announced that he would sign the declaration at six the next morning. And so, in the presence of many illustrious guests, including members of the clergy, his niece read out the two-page document, he signed it, and it was immediately dispatched to Rome. An hour later Talleyrand received the king and queen of France, and in accordance with the correct protocol, presented all those in attendance to them, and died that same afternoon. But when the document reached Rome, it was found to be far from what was expected, and highly inadequate as a confession of his sins. If Talleyrand had lived two or three days longer, he would have had to sign a far more severe act of contrition. But it was too late—he died after receiving the last sacraments, "in the bosom of the Roman Catholic Apostolic Church"—as he wrote in the first sentence of his will. For a long time his confession, so masterfully synchronized with the time of his death, lay on the desk of Pope Gregory XVI, who decided not to call it into question publicly. Then it suddenly vanished and has never been seen again in the Vatican archives.

Would we too, like Talleyrand, want to know the date of our final hour? Would we wish to be able to see an hourglass showing how much sand has already flowed from our life and when the final grain will fall? Raphael, the hero of Balzac's novel *The Wild Ass's Skin*, had this knowledge; he entered life just as Talleyrand was preparing to leave it. One night by the Seine an ancient antiquarian sorcerer gave him a piece of tanned wild ass's skin, which fulfilled all his desires. Stamped on it he made out the mysterious inscription "Every wish will diminish me and diminish thy days." By the end of the novel the talisman is as thin as tissue paper, and Raphael is stricken with extreme terror. He is paralyzed, unable to move; as he stifles all his desires and cravings, "he renounces life in order to live." We are usually spared this fear. If death doesn't come suddenly, its forecast usually reaches us late in the day. Otherwise we'd be unable to bear the thinning air and the growing emptiness as life runs out, and we might even be ready "to pre-empt the final blow."

There is no room for death in today's world, which has gone mad with the idea of eternal youth. Despite being a long way from discovering an elixir of youth, we have already driven death from our thoughts, beyond the range of our consciousness. We deny it the right to exist. We don't talk about death, and we never speak its name, like children who are sometimes afraid to say a particular word for fear of summoning the unwanted item into existence. Still blank, incomplete death certificates are stamped: "Invalidated." We even deprive our cemeteries of an identity; they look like ordinary fields, where we set up rows of graves.

This wasn't always the case. In the Middle Ages and the centuries that followed, death was our constant companion. There were reminders of it everywhere: epidemics, public executions, and funeral processions that passed through towns and villages several times a day. Death was always appearing in picaresque tales, fairground theater shows, monastic teachings about "a goodly death," learned debates, and essays. Awareness of the fact that we shall all die was not subject to erosion. Being "doubly at home"—on earth and in heaven—man knew that the road to the higher home, where Someone was waiting for him, led through death, "the final climb up the rocky chimney stack." Nor was the fact that the end was nigh kept hidden from the dying man; he was fully aware of it and embraced his approaching death, as if he'd already been through the experience before. The act of death was man's self-fulfillment.

There are many accounts of the death of Chopin, which conflict in the details. In the final months it became much harder for him to breathe, and he suffered greatly. Although he was now bedridden at home, he was surrounded by a swarm of people. "All the great Parisian ladies regarded it as de rigueur to faint in his room, where there was also a crowd of draughtsmen, hurriedly sketching him," wrote the opera singer Pauline Viardot. The great Polish poet Cyprian Norwid saw him at the time in the glory of the beauty of ancient times: "The artist's sister sat by him, amazingly like him in profile . . . , in the shade of a deep curtained bed, leaning on pillows and wrapped in a shawl, he was very beautiful, just as ever, with something complete, something monumentally clear-cut about his most ordinary, everyday gestures."

In mid October 1849 his old friend, the one-time insurgent, now Father Aleksander Jełowicki, came to visit him, heard his confession, and administered the last rites. His death agony lasted for three more days and nights. A few hours before he died he asked Delfina Potocka to sing for him. A beautiful woman and a superb artiste, she was to sing songs that included the hymn to the Virgin Mary by Alessandro Stradella, to which healing powers were ascribed. Delacroix said he never heard anything as beautiful as her singing in his entire life. In his final hours Chopin "still found the strength to say a loving word to each person present, and to comfort his friends." He asked his fellow musicians to play nothing but good music. "Do it for me—I'm sure I'll hear you—it'll give me pleasure." He died on 17 October, at two in the morning, and in time-honored fashion addressed his final words to his mother.

So departed the man who came to us "from the land of Mozart, Raphael, and Goethe—his true motherland was the imaginary kingdom of poetry." But it cannot always have seemed as if the angels had come down from heaven to escort him on his final journey. Pain, torment, and suffering must have been far more terrible in those days. They ran their course right there by the open curtain, in full view of a lucid onlooker—the sufferer's consciousness. That was the case until only just over a decade ago. Nowadays we either die suddenly, or sedated with drugs, or unconscious after weeks and weeks of struggling for life in intensive care, or finally after months of *vita vegetativa,* a cabbagelike existence.

She is thirty-eight. Her breathing and heartbeat stopped at dawn during a short, violent asthma attack. Resuscitated at home by the paramedics, she has never regained consciousness, though her lungs and heart got going half an hour after she was brought to the hospital. Two months of treatment in intensive care go by. Although she's breathing on her own and her heartbeat is steady, she shows no response to any sort of stimulus, and all her reflexes are suspended. Her brain cortex—as seen in magnetic resonance—is disappearing and has shrunk to half its size. Her husband and two daughters are at her bedside every day. They say she can sense their presence and answers them by fluttering her eyelids. The nurse says nothing.

She has a milky complexion and a pretty face, in a frame of golden red curls. Her face takes on various expressions of an extremely emotional shade. Feelings run across it and come to a sudden stop, like masks frozen for minutes on end, whole quarters of an hour. Unusually meaningful, with a powerful force of expression, they're like a whole school of emotions for actors. Morning: a mask of extreme despair, with no tears or crying, shocking in its deathly silence. Afternoon: a mask of laughter—the face is flushed with happiness and adoration. This face is laughing, again without making a sound. It's like the Cheshire Cat, I think: she's not there any more—all that's left is her smile.

That evening I go to say good-bye to her. Early the next morning they're taking her to the hospice. Her husband and her younger, ten-year-old daughter are at her bedside. What about the older one? She's taking her school matriculation exams next year. What's she going to be? "An actress," replies the younger one, "and nothing else, even if she has to take her exams ten times over!"

If resuscitation is performed in time, and the cause of heart failure has not proved irreversible, it is possible to restore life. Where have the resuscitated patients been in the meantime? What did they see? These questions fire our imagination so greatly that some people see answering them as a chance to decipher the dualism of body and soul. They are the ones who ask: how can it be possible to be fully aware, to have an out-of-body experience in a state of clinical death, when the brain isn't functioning and the electroencephalogram is showing a flat line, without the tiniest little wobble? The trouble is, no one knows if the impressions described by the patients really occurred to them while their brain had stopped working, or as they were gradually regaining consciousness.

There are two things to say. First, impressions of this kind are a rarity. Not a single one of the almost one hundred patients saved from clinical death whom I have spoken to soon after resuscitation has ever mentioned them to me. In a long list from ten Dutch hospitals, covering some three hundred and fifty patients, only 15% reported any sensations at all. They were limited to statements such as "I knew I was dying," "I was going down a tunnel," "I was aware of a light," "I saw a sky blue landscape," "I met some friends who are dead," or "my whole life passed before my eyes." Second, in the first few weeks after resuscitation the percentage who have something to say is close to zero, but it grows with the passage of time. Some people reckon the patients are embarrassed to mention such paranormal sensations, but we cannot rule out the possibility that they start telling and believing in their story only after hearing similar tales from people who've been resuscitated earlier.

Strange states of existence, somewhere in between life and death, were a source of worry for the romantics, who tried to get through to the world of the dead or the semidead. Edgar Allan Poe often refers to them in his stories, as did Chateaubriand before him. In

Memoirs from beyond the Grave he describes how people deterio-
rate before death, "the transformation of the living into specters,
which they may have been long since anyway," and also the way
they "evanesce and dissolve into thin air." He sees "how before our
very eyes they evaporate into nonexistence." Chateaubriand
sensed the spectral nature of our existence and had more to say
about it than most patients have after being resuscitated. There
have also been cases of exceptional recoveries after years of living
in a state of unconsciousness. Oliver Sacks described the awaken-
ing of creatures that have been in a deep coma for decades, dreaming a ghastly nightmare that they'd been turned to living stone,
imprisoned in the fortress of their own bodies, "in a prison with
windows but no doors."

However, no one can match Plato's Er, the son of Armenius,
who opens Juliusz Słowacki's epic poem *King-Spirit* with the line
"I, Her the Armenian, was lying on the pyre. . . ." He was killed in
battle, and "on the tenth day, when the dead, by now decomposed,
were taken up for burial, his body was found to be perfectly sound.
He was taken home, and on the twelfth day, as he was lying on the
funeral pyre, ready for burial, he came to life again. And having
come to life, he told people what he had seen in the place where he
had been." Er's sentences acquire harmony from the singing of the
Sirens, the Spindle of Necessity turns, the Fates bustle about, and
we hear Ananke, though none of us can see her face.

In the age of romanticism people were afraid of lethargy, apparent death that could not be distinguished from the real thing.
Dead bodies laid out in the mortuary were connected to the un-
dertaker's house by an ingenious system of bells, in case death
turned out to be only apparent, if a dead person moved or got up.
Nicholas Chopin was afraid of being buried alive; all his life he
kept coming back to the subject in letters to his son Frédéric, beg-
ging him to make sure his body was cut up before burial.

Some people fake death to find out how their relatives really
feel about them, or to play on their emotions. In Molière's last

play, *Le malade imaginaire*, the hero tests his family's feelings by
pretending to be dead and thus reveals his wife's greed and his
daughters' love. During the difficult era just after the war, a family
in Wrocław decided to stage the grandmother's death to swindle
the money for the funeral out of their relatives in America. They
ordered a photographer, stood around the bier deep in mourning,
holding lighted candles, and in the silence began to list the relatives for whom copies of the photograph of the dead woman
would have to be made. The count was interrupted by the grandmother, who called out from her coffin: "And one for me!" Apparently the photographer jumped out of the window.

Nowadays death has an exact definition. Whole companies of
doctors, lawyers, neurobiologists, and philosophers have worked
on it. In their efforts to get it right they have tried to match the
precision of mathematicians. In any case, though far from being a
mathematical abstraction, the object they were trying to define
demanded a total lack of ambiguity, in view of sudden advances in
transplant surgery. The recently published story of events surrounding the first heart transplants is a good illustration.

On 3 December 1967 the whole world waited for news from
Cape Town as Christian Barnard removed the heart of a male patient, destroyed by arteriosclerosis, and replaced it with the heart
of a woman killed in an accident. The operation was determined
by a "bold step": the dying woman was hooked up to a respirator
but was given no chance of survival, so Barnard switched it off. As
soon as her heart stopped, he opened her rib cage and took it out.
In the next-door operating theater music began to emerge from a
set of speakers. It was Ravel's *Bolero,* and as it played, the second
team of surgeons opened the recipient's rib cage. They operated
under the spell of this single, nostalgic theme, constantly repeated, returning in a crescendo of color, in an unvarying rhythm.
The first heart transplant patient lived for almost three weeks, but
a few days before he died Barnard performed a second transplant,

modifying his surgical technique. This time the donor was a young man, brought to the Groote Schuur hospital because of a sudden, massive brain hemorrhage. The operation could not start without a diagnosis of death, but the patient was showing signs of life; he still had residual neurological reflexes. Although he could feel the cardiac surgeons breathing down his neck, the head of the internal medicine ward refused to sign the death certificate. At that point he heard one of the transplant team, though not Barnard, say: "God, Bill, what sort of a heart are you going to give us?" The next morning the patient's state of unconsciousness had intensified, the reflexes had disappeared and the transplant went ahead. The recipient, a Dr. Philip Blaiberg, lived for eighteen months. This success paved the way for regular heart transplants.

Christian Barnard was the not the only brilliant expert prepared to carry out transplants. But others, including the American surgeons under whom he studied, were held back by fear of removing a patient's heart without being sure if he were still alive or not. How can you tell? The boundaries of death were not clearly delineated in those days. "Brain death," which nowadays is a crucial element in the diagnosis of death, was still unheard of. Barnard was extremely brave and determined, ready to take the consequences of his action. His "bold step" opened a new era. In the United States almost twenty-five thousand heart transplants are now performed each year. In 75% of them the average life span after the operation is more than five years. It is hard to think of a better example of how effective this treatment can be than the case of a petite, forty-two-year-old American woman called Kelly Parkins, who eight years after her transplant climbed up and down the Matterhorn, unaccompanied by a doctor; the peak is 4,478 meters high, "challenging even for mountaineers in prime health, because it is exposed and there are no resting places."

Recognizing a portent of death or being aware of its onset can release creative power. Two eminent twentieth-century Poles, the psychiatrist Antoni Kępiński and the philosopher Father Józef Tischner, both wrote their best books while bedridden with terminal illness. Both knew perfectly well that the clock had started to tick, and their days were already numbered. At this point in life many of us seem to feel a need to understand ourselves, discover the truth about ourselves, and find life's message. "God speaks to each of us . . . ," wrote Rilke, "before he's formed us." These words echo inside us, although we cannot hear them, because they are hidden by our own amnesia. Their music has been stifled, and with it their meaning. We start looking for life's message only as it runs toward its end. We try to catch it, note by note, in order to hear our own leitmotif, gifted to each of us as individuals.

In 1750 Johann Sebastian Bach reached the age of sixty-five and was seriously ill. He could feel his strength leaving him. On top of that an eye operation had been a failure. He spent the final months in bed, writing, or rather dictating, his peerless work *Art of Fugue*. Never since has this musical form reached such heights. In the third part of the last fugue he introduced a new theme, consisting of four notes corresponding to the four letters of his surname: B-A-C-H (according to German pitch names, where B stands for B flat and H for B). It was unusual to have the sort of name that could be translated into notes (for example, if you tried transferring my name to the musical scale it'd be completely impossible, as only two of the nine letters correspond to notes!). Apparently a manuscript survived on which Carl Philipp Emanuel Bach wrote: "In the course of this fugue, at the point where the name B.A.C.H. was brought in as countersubject, the composer died." According to another version, his state of health prevented him from developing the theme. He still managed to dictate the final prelude and the chorale, briefly regained his sight, and died in a fit of apoplexy ten days later.

Bach must have been familiar with the Roman aphorism *Nomina sunt omina*—"Names are omens." Was there a message hidden in his "musical" name? If so, no one, before him or after, more capable of extracting all the hidden meaning from such a simple musical theme has ever lived. Was he in time to see it? Or hear it? Did he die like Asclepius, the moment he tried to overstep the bounds of human existence?

X. CHIMERA

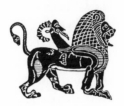

Modern immunology was born when Louis Pasteur made an accidental discovery, from which he managed to extract a general law of biology: a microbe can be weakened so that it loses its pathogenic properties but retains its capacity to stimulate resistance. Pasteur called this phenomenon "vaccination" in honor of Edward Jenner and his *vaccinae*. Soon after, a great show took place. Hundreds of doctors, veterinarians, farmers, and journalists descended on the small town of Pouilly le Fort to watch Pasteur inject lethal doses of anthrax into some sheep, goats, and cows that he had vaccinated in advance. All the animals survived. "From then on," wrote Pasteur's colleague Émile Roux, "there were no longer any skeptics, but only admirers."

Zoonosis—when an infection is transmitted to man from animals—caused by anthrax has practically disappeared from the face of the earth. In the entire twentieth century only eighteen cases of infection were recorded in the United States, transmitted by means of inhalation, among leather tanners. For historical purposes, strains of the bacteria have been preserved in Atlanta and

Novosibirsk. No one gave the extinct cattle disease a second thought until those memorable days in autumn 2001, when envelopes started being distributed by mail containing a highly volatile white powder. In two grams of it, sent by letter to Senator Tom Daschle, there were several billion anthrax spores one to five microns in size. Someone had given them the properties of an aerosol substance, sticking them together with silicon crystals that are easily airborne. No one could be surprised at the panic that gripped the United States. The country was not prepared to inoculate all its citizens against anthrax. Administering such a large number of inoculants was out of the question, on top of which their quality was a cause for doubt, because there had never been a need to conduct this sort of vaccination program before. A new word appeared on the front pages of the newspapers and on the television screens: bioterrorism. Fears of a much more terrible poison made from a bacillus of botulism toxin arose. These fears were fully justified. In the 1990s when the UN conducted weapons inspections in Iraq they found nineteen thousand liters of botulism toxin stockpiled by Saddam Hussein; he had already had some of it loaded into warheads and missiles.

Even more than they fear anthrax and botulism, people have started being afraid of a return of smallpox. Since the 1950s it has been hunted down in the remotest corners of the world, wherever it has made its presence felt, and it has been completely eradicated, which is an extraordinary achievement. How was it done? By means of a vaccination, invented by Edward Jenner, that cut its route of transmission.

Long before Jenner, however, a different kind of inoculation was being practiced in China and Abyssinia, known as variolization. Lady Mary Montagu, wife of the British ambassador in Constantinople, meant to introduce it into Europe. In 1717, in a letter to her friend she wrote: "Today I am going to tell you a thing that I am sure will make you wish yourself here." After describing variolization she ended her letter: "I am a patriot enough to take pains to bring this useful invention into fashion in England and I should not fail to write to some of our doctors very particularly about it, if I knew any one of them that I thought had virtue enough to destroy a considerable branch of their revenue for the good of mankind!" In variolization, which Lady Montagu found so fascinating, matter from inside a sick person's smallpox pustules or a powder made by crushing the scabs they form is injected under a healthy person's skin. The disease develops, but generally has a much easier course than smallpox contracted the natural way, leaving behind an immunity to severe smallpox. However, this was not the rule, fatalities were not exceptional, and Lady Montagu failed to infect the British with her noble dreams.

It was Edward Jenner, a country lad who lost both his parents at the age of five and was a pupil of the local barber before leaving for London, who in 1796 made a discovery that two hundred years later led to the very first disappearance from the face of the earth of one of the most dreadful diseases to haunt mankind. Jenner noticed that milkmaids in the countryside had pockmarks on their hands, but never on their faces. When he asked one of them about it, she replied: "I can't catch human smallpox because I've had the cowpox." Jenner realized that to immunize a person against smallpox there was no need to inoculate him with real smallpox—it would be enough to use cowpox (*variola vaccina*), a common cattle disease that ran its course mildly and was never fatal. In a famous experiment he injected a small boy with an extract from the pustules of a cow suffering from cowpox. Soon after, he did it again with an extract from a human smallpox pustule—and the boy did not contract smallpox. Repeated on hundreds of people, the vaccination always produced the same, unmistakably favorable result. Less than two hundred years later no one on earth was ill with smallpox.

After the World Health Organization's triumphant announcement that smallpox had been totally eradicated, inoculations were suspended in the 1980s. Why bother to immunize against a nonexistent disease? Only the recent chapter in the history of anthrax, dated autumn 2001, has prompted us to think the same thing could happen with smallpox, only much nastier, far more terrible.

Somewhere deep down, dormant within us lies the memory of pandemic disease. The Black Death, leprosy, smallpox, tuberculosis, and influenza have let their mark on the history of mankind. The plague, also known as the Black Death, erupted in 1347 in Manchuria and immediately devoured over ten million Chinese. Then it appeared in Italy and spread like wildfire, engulfing city after city across Europe. According to conservative estimates, in a two-year period it killed one-third of the inhabitants of Europe, in other words, about thirty million people. No one understood the cause of the illness, but they knew it was passed on through contact with the sick, so people barricaded themselves in against infection at monasteries in the mountains or sought refuge deep in the woods. The cities and villages were deserted. On the roads thousands of people pressed ahead, trying to escape. Deserted ships wandered the seas like phantoms once their entire crew was dead. There was no salvation. Death came in three days flat, sometimes in a matter of hours after the symptoms appeared: paralyzingly painful headaches and blistering swellings on the body, which was rapidly covered in dark blotches that turned black, the mark of internal hemorrhages. Believing they had to appease God's anger, people everywhere started practicing zealous piety, and a penitential mood came over them, "from top to bottom —from the benighted populace to the scholars and princes." Those who escaped death did not stop feeling deeply depressed. Until suddenly, after causing so much devastation, the pestilence began to quieten down and, as so often in the past, it disappeared, remaining only in the memory of the survivors. But their enjoyment of life was always under threat, because they knew that "the plague bacillus never dies . . . and that perhaps the day would come when, for the bane and the enlightening of men, it would rouse up its rats again and send them forth to die in a happy city."

Tuberculosis had Europe in its grip for almost two hundred years. Chopin, who according to Hector Berlioz "spent his whole life dying," although that was obviously an exaggeration, suffered a relapse in Palma, Majorca, "despite a temperature of 18 degrees, roses, oranges, palm trees, and figs." At the end of November 1835 he wrote to Julian Fontana: "Of the three most eminent doctors on the entire island, one sniffed what I'd spat, another tapped where I'd spat from, and the third felt and listened to how I spat. One said I've died, the second that I'm dying, and the third that I will die." A fortnight later he was at Valldemosa, an old Carthusian monastery in a wild, isolated valley, after being forced to leave Palma because the local people were terrified of his illness.

What action could doctors take, when they had no idea what was causing the illness? Fifty years later Robert Koch identified the tuberculosis bacillus, and soon after, Wilhelm Conrad Röntgen's discovery of x-rays made it possible to observe the stages of its invasion into the lungs as they became calcified and then fibrous, all the way to their lacunary collapse, which ended in a fatal hemorrhage. There were still no drugs to treat it. People tried to run away from consumption, higher and higher into the mountains—in Poland they went to Zakopane, and in Switzerland to Davos. Europe was covered in a network of sanatoriums. The treatment was based on spending many hours each day lying on open-air terraces. "We have to rest, always lying at rest . . . we live horizontally," says Joachim to Hans Castorp in *The Magic Mountain*. Lying down was supposed to bring salutary mountain air into the collapsing lungs. Polish poet Jerzy Liebert (1904–1931) went to a sanatorium in Bukovina in search of that sort of air and wrote in his *Fir-Tree Lullaby:*

> A scrap of life still rattles away
> Though his lungs are all spat out . . .
> It's just another summer's day
> For the consumptive by the Pruth.
>
> With every day of bright July
> The scent of the fir-trees grows sweet,
> But even the fir-trees are a lie,
> And the air is pure deceit.

The hot weather and the social flirting lent tone to life at the Berghof sanatorium in Davos, where Thomas Mann's wife Katya underwent a cure. However, most of the doctors' efforts were futile, and the patients kept dying like flies. If someone died toward evening or at night, their bodies were sent down to Davos from the sanatorium, which was on the Schatzalp mountain above the town, on bobsleds via a snow chute, because activating the electric railway was very expensive.

It is generally accepted that the tuberculosis epidemic was defeated by streptomycin, which was brought into therapy almost fifty years after Katya Mann's treatment at Davos. Streptomycin really did deal the final blow, but the epidemic had started to retreat many years before it was discovered. The reasons were identified as a better diet, improved public sanitation, and isolating the patients in sanatoriums. Yet why did the number of victims dying of tuberculosis in England and Wales in the Victorian era decrease much faster than the number of people carried off by cholera or dysentery? If better sanitation was not the reason, was it perhaps that "other factors, principally natural selection, played a role"? Perhaps by attacking young people who were susceptible to it, it killed them before they could have children, and as a result, in the next few generations the number of people susceptible to infection by the tuberculosis bacillus decreased. Not everyone finds these arguments convincing. The real reason, still not identified, must be different, but seeing the shadow cast by coming events, the spirit of the epidemic, whose name was always spoken in hushed tones, began to withdraw by itself.

For our grandparents' generation the pandemic illness was influenza (also known as "the Spanish flu," though it originated in Asia). It ran around the globe in 1918, but even half a century later the memory of it stirred alarm. In 1976 when flu caused by a swine virus erupted among the soldiers at Fort Dix, New York, President Ford immediately allocated $450 million to "vaccinate every man, woman and child in the U.S.A." There were all manner of problems with the inoculation, but luckily the epidemic never materialized.

Some medical historians and epidemiologists have hypothesized that the 1918 influenza, like most pandemics, began in China. Others present evidence that it started in Kansas, jumping from one army camp to another, into cities, and then spreading to Europe via troopships. However, the virus could well have emerged from "the gas-ridden, overcrowded trenches and nearby hospitals of already ruined Europe, filled with enough pigs, chicken and ducks to feed two million troops each day." Spain was not more affected by influenza than any other European country, but it was neutral in the war, and unlike the British, French, or German press, its newspapers were not censored and were therefore full of reports about the spread of the epidemic. This caused the name of the disease to be linked with this particular country.

Influenza carried off soldiers and other young men and wiped whole villages and towns off the face of the earth at opposite ends of it. Before fading away in 1920, it managed to kill more people than any other outbreak of disease in human history. The plague that hit Europe in the 1300s killed a far larger proportion of the population—about one-third of the entire continent—"but in raw numbers influenza killed more than plague, more than the First World War, more than AIDS today." The lowest estimate for the death toll is twenty million, but nowadays many epidemiologists believe that influenza is likely to have caused at least fifty million deaths worldwide, and possibly as many as one hundred million.

In 2001 a detailed analysis of the influenza virus was conducted, using samples taken from the corpses of three people killed by the epidemic in 1918. One of them was an Inuit woman, preserved after death in the Alaskan ice. The virus turned out to be a chimera, a cross between the swine fever virus and a human flu virus. Its identifying hallmark, located on the cell membrane, as if on a car windshield, was derived from the human and the swine virus in equal parts. That was why, after entering the human body, it was invisible to the immune system, which was completely unprepared for such an encounter. An encounter with a chimera—a mutant in a cloak of invisibility, invading us at will, blocking our defenses, and destroying its host at lightning speed.

In Greek mythology the Chimera was the daughter of Typhon and Echidna. What a family it was! While Zeus was busy philandering on earth, Typhon—a primitive, evil creature—rose up against him. His enormous bulk stretched between heaven and earth and his one hundred bestial heads, surrounded by a thousand coils of squirming snakes, reached all the way to Olympus. The gods fled in terror to Egypt, where they changed into birds and animals and hid in the desert. Typhon was a step away from conquering Zeus, who in the final struggle tore Mount Etna from its roots and crushed the colossus with it. Echidna, mother of the Chimera, was a repulsive sea monster. The Chimera's siblings included Cerberus, the three-headed hellhound with a hundred snake's tails; the terrible Nemean lion that was killed by Heracles;

the swamp-dwelling Lernaean Hydra; and the Sphinx that tyran-nized Thebes. Homer described the Chimera as "lion-fronted and snake behind, a goat in the middle." So it had a lion's head, belching fire from its jaws, the torso and limbs of an enormous goat, and the tail of a snake. This monster ravaged and scorched the land until it was killed by Bellerophon, who came flying on the winged horse, Pegasus, the epitome of high flight and free-dom, the complete antithesis to the Chimera. As a mongrel hy-brid, the Chimera was at odds with the world's order by its very existence. It went against the laws of nature. It was clearly a made-up creature, "a bastard of the imagination," something so unbelievably hideous that it had to be unreal. As the years went by, its name became synonymous with delusion, fantasy, and hal-lucinations—until it materialized thousand of years later, thou-sands of kilometers from Greece.

Preparations are underway to be ready for the next flu epidemic. More than twenty-five years have passed since the last one to de-stroy half a million human beings. The world is now covered in a network of national laboratories. They collect samples from pa-tients, conduct a preliminary analysis, and send them on to four referral centers, where a detailed appraisal is performed, looking for particularly dangerous strains that could be the source of an epidemic. Soon a single central laboratory will be established that will increase the number of tests at least ten times over. It will fo-cus on automated analysis of the genes of a virus, which can easily change and undergo mutation. The effectiveness of this sort of procedure was proved during the most recent epidemic, which happened in the twenty-first century and caused atypical pneu-monia, defined as "severe acute respiratory syndrome," or SARS. The disease hatched out in a southern province of China before spreading into the neighboring regions and countries. In March 2003, when outbreaks occurred in Southeast Asia, North America, and Europe, the World Health Organization announced a "global alert." About 10,000 people fell ill worldwide, of whom 850 died. By the end of March 2003 the virus had been isolated, and two months later its entire genome had been deciphered. In July 2003 the epidemic was regarded as defeated and the alert was called off. The cause of the disease turned out to be a virus that had a distinct halo of spikes, placing it in the family of coronaviruses. Genome analysis has proved that the SARS virus cannot have been generated by the combination of a human and an animal coronavirus, or two different animal ones. The SARS virus might originally have lain dormant in animals that rarely come into contact with humans, rather than domestic animals. The emergence of SARS in southern China could also be linked to culinary habits. The southern Chinese eat wild game meat as a delicacy; to satisfy this demand, various kinds of wild animal are hunted or raised in captivity. All sorts of live creatures, including civets, raccoons, dogs, sea creatures, wild birds, and domestic birds are to be found squashed in cages, scrambling over each other at the markets, and could well be the source of a newly emerging disease that is infectious to human beings.

Controlling the SARS epidemic was an outstanding achievement of international cooperation. The hardest task is the rapid mass production of vaccinations. Currently, from recognition of a new, virulent strain to developing a vaccination about half a year goes by—a very long time if measured in terms of an epidemic. Enormous efforts are being made to shorten that time and to produce the vaccination against the Chimera more quickly when it sets in—it's a task on the scale of Bellerophon's. The pessimists claim it cannot be done. The optimists remind us that we've already managed to smother the Chimera once before. Finally the fantasists—after all, you need some imagination to fight a monster that first hatched out in the imagination—are already considering the advantages of possessing a nontoxic virus. Sheep and pig hybrids are born nowadays, as a result of genetic engineering, that produce human proteins to cure human diseases. If—say the fantasists—you were to mutate a chimera virus the right way, then in view of its potency and vehemence you could put it to good work. . . . Even so, a little more time will have to pass before mentioning the Chimera implies the epithet "beast of burden."

XI. AFTER
THE GENOME

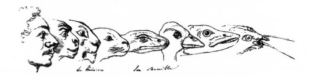

Unarguably, biology's greatest achievement has been to interpret exactly how inheritance works. What an amazing thing it is! Each organism contains instructions on how to create its successor within the capsules of its gametes. These instructions are passed on to the fertilized egg cell, inside which they are gradually disclosed, until the descendant is born. Over the past 150 years biologists have discovered that the way these instructions are passed on is controlled by strict laws, and that they are hidden deep within the nucleus of the cell like jewels in a strong room. They are in the form of a thread—of DNA—and are written in a special code, like a recipe for the shape of an organism and all its functions. The way inheritance works is astounding, and surprisingly universal. DNA sequences tell us how each living creature on our planet is put together from the tiniest building bricks —whether it's a snail or a pine tree, a whale or a beetle, a fly or a human being. These instructions can be translated into a digital code, stored on a computer, and analyzed.

A few years ago we knew only little bits of the information written in DNA. Our success in deciphering those bits, those individual genes, suggested a wild but very exciting idea: what if we "went for broke"? What if we were literally to interpret the entire DNA code, letter by letter? In 1995 it was done for a single-cell organism, a microbe called *H. influenzae.* Three years later it was done for a tiny, transparent worm made up of 957 cells, *Caenorhabditis elegans.* In March 2000 the entire DNA of the fruit fly, *Drosophila melanogaster,* was deciphered. For a whole century this insect had been the subject of continuous intensive genetic research. We know an incredibly large amount about how it inherits its features, and as the language of DNA is universal, the fruit fly's code was bound to help us make sense of human DNA. It could act as a sort of Rosetta stone, but for that we would need a second code, the human one, in order to put the two texts side by side — like on the Rosetta stone, which has Egyptian hieroglyphics next to a Greek translation. The human DNA hieroglyphics, the most important code of all, were obtained just over a year later. In 2001 all three billion letters of human DNA, from A to Z, were deciphered, published, and posted on the Internet. If all the letters were printed out in the font used in this book and put in a straight line, it would stretch from Warsaw to Montreal. The entire DNA contained in a cell is called the genome. Thus, in the third millennium we have started to talk of "medicine since interpreting the genome," or postgenomic medicine.

Let's imagine three billion beads strung on a thread. The beads are in four colors, each corresponding to the letters of the genetic code. Let's put two strings of beads from two different people next to each other. At first sight they're the same, but if we take a closer look we can see that once in every five hundred a single bead is of a different color. Medicine is starting to attach increasing importance to these discreet differences, because they may be able to explain why an individual is susceptible to certain illnesses, or why he responds to one particular drug rather than another. This has been demonstrated in the case of people who are prone to Alzheimer's disease, and also pulmonary embolisms. Quite often these subtle changes have no biological significance, and in most cases we still don't understand them at all.

The variability of individual nucleotides (or letters) of the genetic code is called polymorphism. This word refers back to the beginning of the world, when things were not yet confined by form or frozen into a single shape. When after a long chase Apollo finally caught Daphne, leaf buds started sprouting from her fingers, and she changed into a laurel tree. However, when the girl he loved changed into water, Alpheus agreed to become water too; "without wanting to be held back by the boundaries of an identity" he was united with his love again. And when he lost his senses at the sight of Leda, Zeus transformed himself into a swan, or in the case of Europa into a snow white bull.

So polymorphism was with us at the very start. The ancient Greeks wondered what had happened to it, where on earth it had got to. If Zeus is looking at us nowadays, he must be smiling with joy as he sees us returning, after all those thousands of years, to the very first myth. And it is not in the surrounding world, but inside ourselves that we are finding polymorphism, which was supposed above all to be a feature of the gods.

To get to the bottom of genetic polymorphism, the world's thirteen biggest pharmaceutical firms recently formed a consortium. Soon after, about five million polymorphisms of an individual nucleotide had been discovered, representing only part of the whole, which probably includes a total of ten million. Why did the pharmaceutical giants pump such a vast amount of money into this enterprise? In the belief that decoding polymorphisms will enable us to individualize medical treatment in the near future. We'll take a look at the genes, see a transposed letter and say:

this patient will respond best to such and such a drug. The treatment will be tailored to fit the patient.

However, it is not proving quite so simple. Although searching for the associations between certain polymorphisms and diseases has led to finding a link of this kind in the cases of diabetes, inflammatory bowel disease, and deep vein thrombosis, the human effort and financial cost incurred are dampening initial enthusiasm. The problem is technical in nature. Even if we decide not to investigate an entire genome and concentrate instead on "susceptibility genes," we would have to perform screening tests on tens of thousands of polymorphisms among thousands of people. To do this, the methods currently available to us would need to increase their capacity by one or two orders of magnitude.

A way around these difficulties has been proposed whereby a set of sequence variants could help to detect associations between a genomic region and a disease. Using this method, information from a relatively small number of sets would capture most of the variations in the genome. The concept seems sound, because genetic variants are copied together, if they are located close to each other. The variations found along chromosomes are structured in "blocks," called haplotypes. We may regard the genome as a mosaic of discrete segments (haplotypes), each with its own unique history and relatedness to different contemporary and ancestral individuals. We humans expanded some fifty thousand to two hundred thousand years ago from a rather small African population. "Thus, from a genomic perspective, we are all Africans, either living in Africa or in quite recent exile outside Africa."

Working in tandem with physicians, geneticists have now embarked on the "HapMap" project. Its aim is to determine the common patterns of DNA variations, that is, the haplotypes. In its scope, the HapMap project has much in common with the Human Genome Project, which sequenced the genome, but while the sequencing project covered 99.9% of the entire genome, the HapMap project will characterize the common patterns within the 0.1% of it where we differ from one another. We are just starting to recognize individual words in a language whose alphabet we only managed to decipher very recently.

The cloning of Dolly the sheep demonstrated that every cell of an organism contains the recipe for recreating the whole animal. The same thing goes for man. However, if we were to take a bird's-eye view of the thread of human DNA, we would see that vast regions of it are obscured by darkness. Thousands and thousands of genes are dormant. Elsewhere the lights are on and they're buzzing away. These clusters of illuminated genes send the signals that control the life processes of the cell and the entire organism. These areas of light and darkness can change, especially in the presence of a disease. Recently we have become able to see them. For example, we take a small tumor from under a patient's skin. Suppose it's a neoplasm, lymph cancer, for instance. We extract the DNA from it, and after preparation we place it on a slide the size of a fingernail. The surface of the slide has been coated in advance in detectors able to identify five thousand genes. The active genes, swirling as if in boiling water, shine on the slide with a bright, phosphorescent light. The dormant ones show up only as shadows. An instrument reads the slide and gives us the names of the active genes. The information gained might have an influence on the diagnosis of the illness and its treatment. This technique is called making a nucleotide matrix and has been compared to the discovery of the telescope, because just like a telescope it reveals the countless multitude, not of stars, but genes. In order to take in this mass of information, digest and understand it, we need special computational methods and new, specialized bioinformatics experts.

The active genes set the machinery of the cell in motion, which creates proteins. Being able to recognize all the human proteins has emerged as the next goal after interpreting the genome. It is an enterprise on an unprecedented scale, compared with which deciphering DNA is child's play. Some people want to understand how proteins are expressed in illnesses. Others are concerned with how they interact, and yet others with the functions that depend on their spatial structure. All of them share the hope of finding drugs that will be activated by the proteins discovered. The first pit stop in the race is at the patents office.

Proteomics, as this line of research is called, is a futuristic event. Robots are silently working away in a labyrinth of multistoried laboratories. Their arms go around in all directions, and despite weighing 150 kilograms they are capable of performing extremely delicate tasks. From the tissues provided they isolate a mixture of proteins and divide them into defined sets. Then they break down each component of a set into small pieces and place them in mass spectrometers. Every second, these machines transmit a recognition signal for the piece being tested, known as its "papillary lines." The supercomputer gradually arranges them into a model of the protein. As a result, in a few hours we get a register of several thousand proteins present in the tested tissue. Until recently it took several years to identify a single one.

It is estimated that we carry in us from two hundred thousand to two million proteins. However, the obstacle to recognizing them is not their number, but their variability. While our genes remain basically unchanged throughout our lives, our proteins are constantly changing, depending on the tissue or organ concerned, our age, or even what we had for breakfast. Proteins are like Proteus (the Greek for "first"), the Old Man of the Sea, one of the most ancient beings to inhabit the mythological universe. For the Greeks he was the archetype of metamorphoses, which fascinated them so much and recurred so often in their mythology. Many people went in search of Proteus, just as they search for protein nowadays, because he had the gift of infallible prophesy. But finding and catching him was extremely difficult, because:

Such was Proteus, changing now into a dragon,
Now into rain, now into fire, now into the color of a cloud.

However, proteomics is not nearly as popular as cloning. It feels as if cloning has only had a short history, and that it burst onto the scene in 1997, the day pictures of Dolly the sheep were published. But it all started 170 years earlier, when the notion that life is inseparably linked with cells was accepted; the nineteenth-century German pathologist Rudolf Virchow developed this idea by saying: "Omnis cellula e cellula" (All cells come from cells). Over the next few decades scientists took a close look at the first cells to develop from an egg cell, and the science of embryology came into being. In 1938 Hans Spemann conducted a "thought experiment," which, as he wrote, "appears at first sight to be somewhat fantastical": what would happen if we were to extract the nucleus from the cell of an adult organism and introduce it into an egg cell which has had its own nucleus removed earlier? Fourteen years would pass before the technique of transferring the nucleus was devised, initially in reptiles, and fifty-eight before Dolly was born. "What is now proved was once, only imagin'd," in the words of William Blake.

Because the nucleus from which Dolly was born came from the cell of a mature sheep (and no one had ever succeeded in cloning from mature cells before, not even from those of a frog), and as it was a mammal that was replicated, some people started imagining that human cloning was just around the corner—it was no longer in the realm of fantasy, like something out of Aldous Huxley's *Brave New World*. But we can sense instinctively that cloning is a threat to our identity. Is the day approaching when I shall stop being unique and exceptional, and I'll come face to face—like Narcissus staring into the water—with a living, breathing reflection of myself? Inheritance will cease to be a lottery—instead it'll be controlled by man. However, the individuality of each one of us is formed not only by the genetic material we inherit, but also by our history, character, and features, all of which shape the environment inside us. My identity would not be altered if I had a homozygous twin with exactly the same genetic material. Identical twins are born at almost the same time and come into a world that is equally open to both of them. Things are different in the case of a clone, which is also called a "later twin." The world can no longer be as open to him; the road has already been mapped out by his begetter. He can see it ahead of him and knows he'll follow in his parent's tracks. His knowledge goes further than that of Raphael in Balzac's *The Wild Ass's Skin*. Raphael knows only the time of his own death, but the clone knows his own fate, as handed down to him. Yet we might wonder whether genetic determinism of this kind hasn't been exaggerated. Is the situation of a "later twin" really the complete opposite to that of a child whose overcaring parents never let him out of their sight and influence his decisions for years on end, often taking them for him?

Nowadays, as we seek the secret of eternal youth, the elixir of life, our gaze turns toward stem cells. It is in them that medicine is placing its highest hopes. They are destined to be the fifth essence, Faust's dream come true, salvation for the Sibyl of Cumae. What exactly are these mythical cells? They are the first cells from which all other specialized cells develop. They give a start to the cells of the muscles, liver, bones, and brain. They are the trunk from which the branches of the tree then grow. Is it any surprise that in the stem cells medicine sees a potential panacea for many of the diseases that plague us, and the ultimate refuge from old age? We can't help imagining that if we were to inject them into a damaged liver, for example, they would change into liver cells and the liver would regenerate. The same thing could happen with other organs, and so the idea of regenerative medicine has been born. There are stem cells lying dormant in most of our tissues and organs, but they are scattered and few in number. There are slightly more, though still not many, in the blood. Their main source, however, is the bone marrow, where erythrocytes, leukocytes, and the other components of the blood develop out of them. From there they can be easily obtained and injected into the heart muscle, for instance.

By mid-2004 an estimated two hundred patients in the world had had cells transplanted into their hearts. Most of them were suffering from severe heart attacks or chronic heart failure. In each case, many millions of cells were injected straight into the heart muscle or via a catheter placed in a coronary artery.

Assessments of this procedure are very optimistic and imply that it helps to improve the muscle's ability to contract. However, we shouldn't forget that so far only a small number of tests have been performed, and that cell transplants are usually combined with revascularization (angioplasty or coronary stenting); it may be completely impossible to distinguish between the beneficial effects of these procedures. Nonetheless, there is enormous enthusiasm and preparations are already underway for a controlled clinical trial, including about four hundred patients, though there is still a lack of resources to carry it out.

How implanted stem cells work to produce their favorable effect is still unclear. Do they undergo transformation into heart muscle cells, like Daphne, who transformed herself into a tree? Or do they fuse with resident muscle cells, "becoming a mermaid, half-woman and half-fish"? They might also get involved in the production of new blood vessels, leading to an increase in the blood supply. Perhaps in the future it will be possible to isolate stem cells from small cardiac biopsies and to expand them in vitro for subsequent clinical use, for example, in the reconstruction of dead or scarred heart muscle following their percutaneous injection. "Stem-cell therapy provides immense possibilities but also problems that have never been accounted before."

The substance that we inject, taken from the bone marrow, is heterogeneous material. If only we had pure stem cells! But of course we do—they are present in the fetus, at the very start of life. It is from those primary, embryonic stem cells that the cells of the heart, liver, brain, and so on, will later develop. In 2004 human embryonic stem cells were obtained for the first time ever, by means of cloning, in Seoul. How was it done? The nucleus was squeezed out of a woman's egg cell and replaced with another nucleus, taken from the cells surrounding and nourishing the egg cell. This nucleus came from the same woman as the egg cell. After that, the right conditions were provided in vitro for the cloned cell to multiply over the next few days, to a stage of about one hundred derivatives. At that point tests were performed proving that the cells formed were indeed stem cells that could generate many different tissues. The experiment ended there.

Critical to the Korean team's success was their collection by means of laparoscopy of 242 egg cells from sixteen young women who agreed to undergo advance hormone therapy that caused them to ovulate excessively. No one had ever succeeded in getting hold of such a large quantity of human egg cells before, though this technique for getting eggs from women's ovaries has been used for years for in vitro fertilization purposes. Who were these women? The original Korean publication describes them as volunteers who took part in the research willingly, without receiving any payment.

The news from Seoul ran around the world like wildfire. The directors of the research team became national heroes, received dozens of invitations to give lectures, and immediately found themselves on *Time* magazine's list of the most influential people in the world. Hordes of journalists descended on their laboratories in Seoul, which were regarded as a proper cloning factory. Scientists from Western countries speak with awe of the phenomenal talents of their Korean colleagues and their total dedication to work, which goes on from 6 a.m. to 10 p.m. every day. When asked what made his team so successful, Woo Suk Hwang replied: "No Saturdays, no Sundays, no holidays." What's he working on now? Cloning cattle that would be immune to mad cow disease, and the recreation of a variant species of the completely extinct Siberian tiger (*Panthera tigris altaica*). He prefers not to be questioned about the medical applications of his work. And yet that is the heart of the matter. The Koreans achieved something that everyone has been debating for several years, professionally known as therapeutic cloning. They succeeded in obtaining human embryonic stem cells, which could soon be injected into patients. If one of the women on whom the above-mentioned cloning procedure was performed were a patient needing an organ transplant, she would not need immunosuppression, which is a routine part of the treatment, because the cloned cells would come from her own body. However, we should not be under any illusions. Therapeutic cloning has set the door ajar for reproductive cloning. In this procedure, blastulas (the developmental stage of a cloned embryo at which the Koreans stopped) would be injected into the woman's uterus, causing her to give birth to a cloned child.

So is the development of biotechnology bound to end in children to order? Reproductive cloning, or in other words experiments aimed at cloning a complete human being, is banned worldwide. The situation with therapeutic cloning for remedial purposes is different. Cells can be sourced from early embryos from the period before they take root in the uterus (called blastocytes). Embryos of this kind are available at infertility treatment clinics (practicing in vitro fertilization), where they are often obtained in excess, as so-called supernumerary embryos. They are either doomed to necrosis, or else are preserved in a frozen state if their parents envisage further pregnancies. The only other way of obtaining embryonic stem cells is to create them by means of cloning.

In Europe, the most liberal legal regime is in force in Great Britain, where both these possibilities are allowed, that is, the use of human embryos to create cell cultures (or lines), and also to create embryos (cloning) for research purposes. In Finland, Greece, Holland, and Sweden creating embryonic lines of stem cells from supernumerary embryos is allowed. In Austria, Germany, France, Ireland, Spain, and Poland the law forbids such research. Yet even if, as in the United States, the government does not allow scientists to obtain stem cells in the research units which it finances (which would result in the destruction of an embryo), private biotechnology firms have no trouble getting round this ban and are now investing tens of millions of dollars in the cloning of human embryonic stem cells, especially since the spectacular success of the Korean scientists.

But cloning really is a highly unnatural form of reproduction and will lead to equally unnatural relations between parents and their children. A cloned child will be at the same time both the child and the twin of the parent from whom it inherits its genes but will have no blood relationship with the other parent at all. That parent will bring up a younger version of his or her spouse. The enthusiasts are already predicting that we're going to take control of the biological side of our nature, no longer leaving it to the blind powers of natural selection. And then we'll be in the "post-human world," where we'll mix human genes with the genes of other species, so in the end we won't know what a human being is any more.

However, do we really have to accept that sort of world under the false standard of freedom? Do we really have to regard ourselves as the slaves of inevitable technical progress? How should we define the border beyond which biotechnology should not be allowed to interfere in the human organism? What do we ultimately want to protect? The essence of our humanity, the heart of our human dignity, and the laws that arise from it? The notion of human dignity, a major theme of the pontificate of John Paul II, is staggeringly topical for us today. The border crossed by Asclepius, whose penalty was to be struck down by a thunderbolt, really does exist, however hard it is for our eyes to see.

The genome is festooned in high-flown metaphors. It has been called the Bible of creation, the Book of Man, a recipe for life, the manual of evolution, nature's code, the Holy Grail, and the language of God. Interpreting the genome has been compared to splitting the atom, men landing on the moon, the achievements of Galileo, Shakespeare, and Rembrandt, and the invention of the wheel. And what has it actually brought us? A lot of surprises.

The number of genes turned out to be fewer than we had thought earlier, and totals about thirty thousand. How can we reconcile this with the wide diversity of proteins, which exceed that number by a long way? Until recently we accepted that one segment of DNA, defined as a gene, contained the recipe for just one single protein. Thus, we used to say that one gene coded for one protein. Since then, the fact that one gene codes for several variants of protein has proved to be the norm. The process involved is universal, occurs during production of mature RNA, and is called splicing.

Genes make up only 1.5% of DNA. They have been compared to oases scattered about the desert. So what exactly is this staggeringly enormous desert? It is made up of tens of thousands of recurring motifs. Some are very simple, built of two letters in tandem, such as CACACACA. Others are incomparably more complicated. Lots of them are mobile, able to move from place to place within a chromosome, and in this regard they remind us of shifting desert sands. There are also virus genomes scattered among them, usually "decayed relics that no longer have the capacity to form viruses." Once upon a time, somewhere in the process of evolution, they must have been incorporated within us. The desert wastes are also filled by elements that regulate the function of the genes, pseudogenes, and "immigrants" (scraps of DNA transferred from microbes, for example).

The desert metaphor does not seem very apt. "The barren desert . . . could be highly fertile research terrain." The genome conceals the enigma of evolution within its structure. It can be compared to "the archaeological excavation of an unknown civilization." Just as in archaeology, what is valuable is hidden among piles of earth.

If the vast majority of the human genome does not code for proteins, why do we need so much DNA? Some scientists have assumed that repetitive DNA elements have no function; they are just useless, selfish sequences that proliferate in our genome. The term "junk" DNA was coined to describe these repetitive elements. Now, however, more and more geneticists are starting to regard the repetitive elements as genomic treasure. These elements interact with the surrounding genomic environment and increase the ability of the organism to evolve. They provide preset motifs for new transcriptional regulatory elements and for rapid rearrangement of the genes. Therefore, repetitive DNA "should be called not junk DNA but a genomic scrap yard, because it is a reservoir of ready-to-use segments for nature's evolutionary experiments."

Many human genes are surprisingly similar to the genes of other multicell organisms. Astonishingly, human beings and mice retain some completely identical genomic segments, even though the two species are separated by at least two hundred million years of evolution. Comparative research into the human genome and that of other living organisms is likely to reveal how evolution works. Will it be able to explain the details of evolution that cause heated arguments or are the cornerstone of some people's instinctive rejection of evolution? They refuse to believe in it, despite the fact that biological evolution is merely one in a succession of links in the great cosmic process of change. It fits logically in the picture of the world drawn by modern cosmology, which is "evolutionary through and through": from the Big Bang, via the synthesis of chemical elements to the birth of the galaxies, stars, planets, and finally living organisms. The attitude of the Apostolic See is also clear, as expressed in John Paul II's celebrated letter to the Papal Academy of Sciences, dated 22 October 1996, which sums it up in the sentence: "The scientific theory of evolution is not at odds with any truth of the Christian faith."

Yet resistance to the theory of evolution continues to exist. It unites "a considerable number of theologians and clergy" as well as "some Christian believers." This is evidenced not only by the fact that "man does not want to accept the truth about his ancestors." It is more often a reaction to the rather obvious "epistemological abuses" of the modern Darwinists, who suggest that science excludes the existence of God.

Reluctance to accept the theory of evolution may also have to do with the language in which it is presented, the metaphors used to describe it. Scientists have a soft spot for metaphors and are often as sensitive to them as poets, even though they create far fewer. Apt metaphors, striking similes, or deliberately ambiguous statements have all contributed to the development of science just as much as rigorous conclusions based on objective data. The language used by the evolutionists rouses spirited objection from Czesław Miłosz:

> The battles among genes, traits that secure success, gains and
>   losses.
> My God, what language these people speak
> In their white coats.

The metaphors used by the neo-Darwinists (though Charles Darwin himself avoided them), came to light in an era when capitalism was flourishing and have been revived in a new form in the past few decades. Richard Dawkins's "selfish gene" has gained the greatest renown. We have started regarding the human body as a carrier of DNA containing a vortex of selfishly disposed genes with one single purpose: to reproduce in the heat of battle. Selfishness, warfare, egoism, ruthlessness, the triumph of the mighty —these words come back time and again in the works of the leading modern biologists. And although they do warn us—once in a while—not to take them too literally, "the disclaimers are brief, and so completely without effect on their surroundings that they have no more force than the tiny warnings on cigarette packets. Like those warnings, they are cancelled by their context."

According to the biologists, in their sphere of science cooperation and joint action are just as common as competition. The survival of life on earth may well depend on keeping a balance between all forms of existence. What's more, animate and inanimate matter are interconnected by a coherent system of two-way exchanges, which prompts us to look at the earth as a whole, as a single living organism. That was how James Lovelock imagined it about thirty years ago, when he created the theory, or hypothesis, of Gaia. In mythology Gaia was one of the first creatures to emerge from Chaos. She was a living organism, with valleys and hills, like enormous limbs. Lovelock's poetic Gaia hypothesis assumes that although organisms compete with one another on a local scale, in the broader perspective their interaction creates an environment that is better adapted and more conducive to life. "Organisms and their environment evolve as a single, self-regulating system." To many people, this idea is too far a departure from Darwin's theory, but adherents of Gaia, whose numbers are growing, believe that it develops rather than contradicts Darwin's version of events.

An equally comforting image, far removed from the ruthless rivalry of individuals, is provided by evolutionary theology. According to this thesis, nature is not just a blind game of chance, nor does it contain a hidden plan of evolution that the Omnipotent Designer wants to impose with ruthless inevitability. Evolutionary theology speaks of God's vision of change, and in this respect it reminds us of modern physics, which talks about "God's mind." God does not determine the widely dispersed conditions of the universe unambiguously, but "makes man His confidant, jointly responsible for the future shape of the work of creation."

As the Bible's description of original sin would already have indicated, evolution could sometimes run away from God's vision. Both these poetical theories, Gaia and evolutionary theology, remain on the sidelines of the main trend of scientific evolutionism. However, the debate over the driving force of evolution never dies down. Some people suggest that Darwin was wrong to emphasize competition and selection as the only forces shaping the origin of species; to their minds it is "cooperation and symbiosis that drive evolution."

The theory of evolution brings chance into our lives, shattering the idea of the world's harmony and coherence. When in autumn 1996 at the Papal Academy of Sciences there was a session devoted to evolution, the debate spread beyond the walls of the Vatican, to the students of Rome, who reacted by producing hundreds of identical placards, featuring a picture of the world with a rocket-shaped capsule zooming skyward away from it. In it sits a severe, tough-looking Darwin, the way we remember him from drawings at school, in a long frock coat, with a neatly trimmed beard. He is going up into the sky, against a horizon made up of the Sistine Chapel fresco that depicts God touching Adam's outstretched hand. Power, as portrayed by Darwin rushing from the earth, is making the firmament split, pushing God's hand away from man.

Is this split the inevitable upshot of automatic, random evolution? Does it bring about "linear time extending infinitely backwards and forwards"? Or maybe chance is not entirely without motives, at which point what a physicist sees at the quantum level and a biologist sees at the level of evolution is chance invading, reality being pervaded by an alien causality that is incomprehensible to us, and yet consistent. Exploring the history of the genome, digging down to its oldest, deepest layers, might one day make these mysteries less obscure.

XII. ALTERATIONS
AND RETURNS

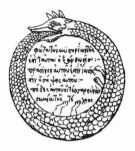

As illnesses come and go, their treatment changes. Take operations for coronary heart disease, for example. Their history goes
back a hundred years. To begin with, the surgeons used to discon-
nect the heart from the control of the nervous system, in an attempt to remove pain and dilate the arteries. There was a wide
range of procedures: cutting the sympathetic nerve branches running to the heart, removing the nerve ganglions situated on the
aorta, or injecting anesthetics into the large clusters of nerve cells
wound around the carotid artery. None of these operations
changed the course of the disease. In the 1930s the rib cage was
opened, the heart exposed and its surface rubbed. The epicardium
was scraped to elicit its inflammatory reaction and prompt the development of new blood vessels. Another deluded hope was that
you only had to cover the heart with the peritoneum and the arteries from this membrane, which has a rich blood supply, would
come running to the rescue of the heart. In a similar way the heart
was brought into contact with the lungs or other tissues capable of
supplying blood rich in oxygen. Later on the arteries close to the

heart were ligated so that blood from them would recede into the coronary circulation. The large pectoral arteries were also sewn directly to the heart muscle. However, the results hoped for were not achieved.

So it is not surprising that when at the end of the 1960s the first reports about a new heart operation appeared they were received with mistrust and incredulity. *Timeo chirurgos et dona ferentes* ("I fear the surgeons, even bearing gifts"), wrote leading cardiologist Charles Friedberg at the time, parodying Laocoon's warning at the sight of the wooden horse under the walls of Troy. Being men of action, the surgeons were not upset by the skeptical comments of their colleagues educated in the humanities. Just as ever, they moved ahead swiftly and noisily. But this time they achieved incredible success. The operation they performed, involving casting bridges of vein across constricted sections of artery, in other words bypassing them, displaced all the other procedures in use before then, becoming the most popular heart operation and one of the most frequently performed operations in general.

Over the years the operations have become less and less traumatic. Just as you can look into a room through the keyhole without opening the door, so nowadays a surgeon can penetrate the heart without opening the entire rib cage through a small hole in its wall—so-called keyhole surgery. Constricted sections of the coronary arteries are also widened by inserting ingenious catheters with tiny inflatable balloons into the heart via a puncture in the femoral artery. At least a hundred such operations are performed in Poland every day. Yet thirty years ago they were completely unheard of. The impressive development of medicine has its price, quite literally—it is expensive, very expensive.

The healthcare systems in the world's richest countries are tottering. At the start of her husband's first presidential term, Hilary Clinton came a cropper over reform of the healthcare system and made no further attempts at reform. The National Health Ser-

vice, for many years the pride of Great Britain, has found itself up
a blind alley because of spiraling costs. Everyone's complaining:
the patients because they're forced to wait months to see a doctor
or to be admitted to a hospital, and the doctors and nurses because
they're overworked, lack job satisfaction and, of course, are badly
paid. In spring 2002 Prime Minister Tony Blair announced revo-
lutionary changes in the British healthcare system, comparing
them in scale to the radical reform of British industry conducted
twenty years earlier by Margaret Thatcher.

The ideology of business is permeating medicine. Politicians, ad-
ministrators and accountants have come onto the scene. "As the
fog of human-resources jargon obscured an emptiness of serious
thought, so mediocrity became the benchmark for running a
health service. Priorities shifted. Quality was eroded by a concern
for quantity . . . . Morale collapsed, cynicism became commonplace," wrote the editor-in-chief of the *Lancet*. It is hard to suspect the average self-possessed Briton, famous for his nerves of
steel, of giving in to a passing mood of panic, especially as similar
words are being loudly voiced on the other side of the Atlantic.

In 2002 the leading American and European medical associations jointly announced a Physician's Charter. "Changes in the
health-care delivery systems in virtually all industrialized countries threaten the very nature and values of medical professionalism," we read in the Charter. It tersely reminds us of the principles
of the profession and sums up a doctor's duties. The feeling that
we're dealing with something very familiar comes over us—we
get a sense of déjà vu. Time for the diagnosis: as we read the
Physician's Charter issued in 2002, we can't help noticing, line after line, that we're running our eyes down the pages of a charter issued 2,500 years ago—the Hippocratic Oath.

Healthcare is being buried under an avalanche of expense. As if
that wasn't enough to cope with, medicine itself is taking on new

obligations. Nowadays it declares that its task is not just to cure illness in each individual case, but to keep society healthy; from concentrating on the individual patient it is directing its attention toward larger groups of people, covering whole communities with prevention. Contact with the doctor is starting to change from occasional to constant, with emphasis on treatment at home or at outpatient centers, not just "being put in the hospital."

So how should a doctor carry out treatment? "Safely, quickly and pleasantly" (*cito, tuto et iucunde*) replied Asclepiades of Bithynia in 120 BC, a successful Roman doctor who eulogized the therapeutic powers of wine. The modern answer would be: According to the principles of evidence-based medicine. In the past decade a particular model of clinical experiment has become well established, especially in drug research. It must be conducted in a "controlled" and a "randomized" manner, "with a double-blind test" (meaning that both the researcher and the person being tested are unaware of whether a drug or a placebo has been administered in a given instance). Only after meeting some rigorous criteria, often involving tens of thousands of patients, and conducting scrupulous expert assessment of the records, the statistical analysis, and the way the conclusions were drawn can the results be recognized as credible, as "substantiated." The procedure is long, costly, and, it has to be said, does not require much imagination. So do we really have to make our lives so complicated? Yes, until we find a better way of answering the question whether a new drug is effective or not, or even whether or not it's better than its predecessors. In this dichotomy between "objective science" and "the subjective truth" medicine declares itself in favor of the former. What's more, as opposed to modern physics, it refuses to brook any subjectivism in clinical drug research. This attitude borders on logical positivism, or the rationalism of the Enlightenment era. Yet in defense of medicine it is only fair to say that in this particular case, in contrast to physics, it has no possibility of using mathematical modeling to illustrate the real world. It also knows well that a doctor conducting research may be susceptible to various influences, not excluding those of the powerful pharmaceutical industry. So it prefers to "blindfold" both him and the patient.

Curiously, medicine likes to don the robes of a science and declares itself to be one, while the exact sciences make no secret of their own doubts about their foundations. The efficiency of mathematical logic was put to the test by Gödel's theorem. Physicists dream of an ultimate theory that would bring together two incongruous, schizophrenically divided worlds ruled by separate laws—the world of classical mechanics, precise and geometric, and the quantum world, indeterminate and probabilistic.

It is fashionable nowadays to talk of "departing from paternalism," of "treating the patient as a partner," or to say that "medical treatment is a matter of negotiation." The patient has a right to expect that his situation, the ways of resolving it, and their pluses and minuses will be clearly explained to him. Thus, the decisions remain in the hands of the interested party—and not in order to comply with the maxim that "the doctor always washes his hands before an operation"! But even after the most discerning, thorough analysis there is always an element of faith in the patient's decision . . .

When Alexander the Great was seriously ill the doctors did not dare to treat him, for fear of losing their heads if he died. Only Philip of Acarnania, the king's doctor and friend, was brave enough to come to his aid and prepare some medicine for him. Just then Parmenio, the most loyal of his courtiers, sent Alexander a letter warning him: "O King, Philip has been bought up by Darius, King of Persia, with the promise of marriage to his daughter, and is coming to poison you." Alexander did not show the letter to anyone, and when Philip came, carrying a goblet full of the prepared medicine, he gave him the letter to read, while at the same time he drank the medicine without showing any fear. And so one drank while the other read, until they were staring into each other's eyes.

This dramatic scene illustrates two medical themes. The first is an uncompromising attitude in fighting an illness—all the doctors went away except Philip. The second is the patient's faith in his doctor. Alexander trusted Philip and didn't believe Parmenio's warning. The doctor strives for that trust, and when he wins it, he can sit and marvel at its power as he says to himself: "Dear patient, if only you knew how colossally ignorant I am, how very impotent; if only you knew how little I know!"

Ignorance is especially burdensome when you can see that despite your best efforts the illness is taking the upper hand and life is fading. But what exactly is life, which it is a doctor's primary duty to preserve? At an international symposium on the definition of life that was held in America, toward the end of the second day of long debates an agreement was reached: "The ability to reproduce—that is the essential characteristic of life." Everyone breathed a sigh of relief, but then a small voice piped up from the back of the room and said: "Then one rabbit is dead. Two rabbits—a male and a female—are alive, but either one alone is dead." Since then hardly anyone has tried to define life in terms of a single characteristic. Recently a renowned Nobel Prize winner adopted a definition based on seven attributes. He called them the pillars of life. To specify each of them he needed a separate column of print. "Living matter and clarity are opposites—they run from one another," wrote Einstein in a letter to Max Born.

A small book by Erwin Schrödinger entitled *What Is Life?* prompted a spirited response. Published in 1944, it was the source of inspiration for successive generations of scientists. Yet it was "neither original, nor up-to-date, nor accurate. It was short on both hard facts and rigorous arguments." Its power to have such an influence actually lay in insinuations. It gave everybody whatever they wanted; no one could really tell, for instance, what Schrödinger had in mind when he wrote: "Living matter, while not eluding the 'laws of physics' as established up to date, is likely to involve 'other laws of physics' hitherto unknown, which, however, once they have been revealed will form just as integral a part of this *science* as the former." The book was full of statements like that one, woven out of a mist that presumably concealed some highly visionary landscapes. All were entitled to their own conjectures, reductionists and antireductionists alike. And so the great physicist, cocreator of quantum mechanics, achieved a success in biology, by applying, as it were, in his own words the uncertainty principle that rules the quantum world—by using "studied ambiguity."

Two great Russians, the poet Joseph Brodsky and the writer Vladimir Nabokov, both compared life to a kind of fabric. At first sight its weft and warp threads interweave in a chaotic manner. But if you look carefully, you can pick out an original pattern: "a capricious line of repetitions, a mysterious theme in an obvious story, zigzags of reflections and echoes." An elaborate drawing, a game of motifs, and a background all come to light in rare moments of revelation, and also when "we cross over to the other shore"—when we die. "Greek mythology," wrote Brodsky, "is the most thoughtful vision of this fabric created by existence, aware that this fabric is torn apart and stained, and that its edges are flapping in the darkness." The writer investigates these rips and stains, and especially the ragged edges that border on darkness, "because darkness is the same sort of fabric too."

We ascribe the extreme difficulties we encounter in attempting to encapsulate life within a definition to its individual uniqueness, so we should not expect science to provide an answer to our question about the essence of life. The realm of science covers recurrent phenomena—a scientific result has to be repeatable in any laboratory. For this to be the case, we need to extract the repeatable essence of each experiment—which is after all a singular event—and purge it of its individual, subjective elements. Only then does it come under the umbrella of science. This strategy has proved extremely effective. In exchange for renouncing individuality, we gain knowledge about the foundations of nature.

However, "nature is rich in exactly these elements where purely mechanical motion predominates. Its richness in this respect falls off noticeably in biology, and all but vanishes in man. Science, by its nature, can have nothing interesting to say about individual human values." The forces that motivate human beings remain outside the realm of science, though that certainly doesn't mean they have to be supernatural; on the contrary, they are often patently obvious. Science is not able to answer questions that start with Why? or What for?—questions "asking about reality at its deepest level." It can reply only to questions beginning with How?—a fact worth remembering nowadays, when science pervades every area of human life, including the spiritual. Along with technology it has become the new religion. We see it as a source of liberation, as well as the satisfaction of all sorts of material needs. We optimistically expect medical science to invent a drug to cure death. We accept it as perfectly natural for science to embrace the realms of ethics and morality. When everything can be measured, talking about the spiritual foundations of things sounds old fashioned, causing the audience at best confusion. Busy with other concerns, science doesn't worry about inner life; modern mass culture is completely ignorant of it and is destroying it. And yet "only in the inner life, as in a broken mirror, do we occasionally catch a glimpse of eternity's small, mobile flame, whatever the mocking (or not) reader may understand this to be," writes the contemporary poet Adam Zagajewski.

Not without reason, many people accuse science of secularizing Western societies. However, before we agree to regard science as the modern religion, before we heap blame on it for our various sore points and misfortunes, let us be aware not only of its powers, but also its limitations, the boundaries of scientific knowledge. Marking out these boundaries is not always going to be easy, but they do exist. Beyond them lie worlds inaccessible to science, the worlds of values, art, faith, and all the other singular, individual phenomena.

When the years start to add up, time goes ever faster and the shadow line is far behind us, we start to feel a longing to understand the nature of the profession that has swallowed up our life. Some artists are overwhelmed by this longing, aching to get through to the mystery of art, which is at the same time the mystery of life. Johann Sebastian Bach sought the answer in a musical motif based on the letters of his name. Picasso's reaction was to isolate himself from the world in his studio near Cannes and search for the mystery of his art in Velázquez's great painting *Las Meniñas*. The heroine of the picture is the fair-haired girl, the little infanta in her stiff crinoline. She is standing in a large room with a mirror reflecting the royal couple, surrounded by ladies-in-waiting, a dwarf, and a nun talking to a man dressed in black in the half-light. On the other side we can see Velázquez in front of a large canvas set on an easel, holding an artist's palette and wearing black court dress and a white ruff. First Picasso painted the same picture in steel gray colors, opening wide the door at the very back of the original scene to let in the light. Then he swooped down on the infanta and the other figures like a fury, breaking them in half and reassembling them, bringing out the eyes, then the hair and the noses, and adding all possible colors. Like Vesalius, he wanted to see what lay inside them, to rip the secret out of their entrails. Just as Bach did for Goldberg, he produced dozens of variations on the theme of the infanta, each one revealing new, previously imperceptible features of her, as she went through as many changes as Proteus. Each painting tried, through metamorphosis, to reveal her hidden essence, to encapsulate the unique nature of art.

Sometimes our own faces are suddenly revealed to us, but we fail to recognize them. That's what happened to Narcissus, who spent his time wandering about the forests and mountains. One day he saw his own face reflected in a pool of spring water and fell in love with it. But the reflection refused to leave the forest pond, so finally Narcissus pined away from unrequited love and died. Some said he was punished by Aphrodite for scorning the love of the nymph Echo. His punishment was failure to recognize himself.

In fact, we are born with the capacity to distinguish ourselves from the rest of the world. This function is performed by the immune system. Billions of its specialized cells reach into the far corners of the body, asking the other cells for a password, which they find written on their surface. If there is the slightest shadow of doubt they mobilize a mighty army to destroy the intruder who has crossed the barrier of what constitutes the "self." In so-called autoimmune diseases the patient's ability to distinguish the "self" from the "nonself" suffers a breakdown. This is the sort of illness that affected Narcissus. In autoimmune disease the body regards its own tissues as something alien and declares war on them. Then the doctor applies strong drugs that intoxicate the immune system and stifle its suicidal effects. We take similar action in transplant surgery—we put spectacles on the immune system to make it see an alien, grafted organ as its own.

What exactly constitutes the self? Let's not ask immunology that question. By digging ever deeper into its complex structures, we are getting to know the mechanisms that separate the self from the nonself. We can make out the passwords on the surfaces of the body's cells, which the immune system patrols ask for, and we can see how they read the cells' ID cards. We are becoming familiar with the connections between the immune system and the nervous system, which lead us to suppose that immune signals from the furthest corners of the body come together within the central nervous system. Thus, we are getting close to answering the question of how we recognize our self, but its essence remains unknown to us. There must be some integral element contained inside it, hence many people associate our self with our consciousness and even seek a material substrate for it within the brain. This issue fascinates nonspecialists and attracts eminent thinkers. The great British mathematician Roger Penrose believes that quantum effects, crucial for the consciousness to come into being, occur within microscopic structures of the brain neurons, so-called microtubules. Francis Crick, codiscoverer of the double spiral of DNA, places consciousness in the network that links the neocortex and the hypothalamus. The arguments of mathematicians and physicists stir the imagination but do not convince everyone. *Ignoramus et ignorabimus,* say the skeptics. How can you localize on the map of the brain something that we are unable to qualify, and that it is surely impossible to define? Aren't we talking about incomparably singular phenomena that elude generalization? Biology and the exact sciences have nothing to say on the subject of consciousness beyond what has already been revealed by philosophy and literature. So the self, the thing that's closest of all, remains the hardest to grasp, even though it is the focal point of our very being, a miniature archeus, "the person within" who rules over us. The mystics, those spiritual masters, also see it as the seat of our pride, constantly demanding recognition, stridently voicing opinions, causing resentment, occupying every thought, and driving most of our emotions. Whatever era they happen to live in, they all recommend "effacing the self," transcending it, and emerging on the other side of our own egotism. These views accord with those of medicine, which accepts them as its own. Its aim lies beyond ourselves, in another, unhealthy person. In order to help him, said John Paul II, "you must give yourself," your own self; you must open up your self for another person. Suffering is also present in the world in order "to liberate the love in man, the disinterested gift of his own 'self' on behalf of other people, people who are suffering." And so medicine concerns perhaps the strongest of human desires—our longing for love, which is usually unfulfilled.

Few people had as strong a sense of his own individuality as Paracelsus, who opened his medical credo with the words "I am different, let this not upset you." At the same time he professed that the doctor would open up to the patient more fully if he remembered to think of the spiritual connection linking all things together that dominates the universe. He regarded the universe as a living creature, within which, on the model of man, the very smallest parts are all interconnected. At the same time Spinoza explained the science of the unity of the universe *more geometrico,* that is, in a precise, mathematical way, coming from axioms to proof of his theorems. Just like the modern Gaia theory, the theories of Paracelsus and Spinoza sound like distant echoes of the beliefs of the ancient Greeks. They saw the world as a living organism. Both Plato and Aristotle, as they gazed at the stars and planets, saw animals, and placed the gods in categories of entities alongside birds, fishes, and terrestrial beasts. They were determined to seek out unity in the world, in the strong conviction that despite appearances everything is imbued with a common, unifying feature, like Ananke's net falling from the sky. And in the myths they created, in one single figure, in one single event, they perceived all the others that it contained.

They firmly believed in the magic of art, which, following the example of the art of medicine, brings *katharsis,* because "art is the conjuration of existence to continue."

Every acutely progressing illness reaches a crisis point. All sorts of defective elements are unloaded amid a storm of symptoms, and the body undergoes a purification, along with an emotional shock.

The patient suddenly senses that the illness is passing, and then feels sure it won't return. Suddenly "you see the world lit differently." Everyday things lie patiently waiting for us to touch them and pick them up—once again the world exists only for us to fill ourselves with its wonders. As in a moment of revelation, "instead of many roles and all manner of purposes, the real meaning of life becomes clear." As we listen to patients who have been through this, *katharsis* becomes plain to see. All the doubts that our minds have swathed it in for centuries slip away. Now it radiates certainty, becoming clear and distinct, like the vision of a new life that briefly appears to the patient the moment he emerges from illness—when he experiences catharsis.

NOTES

RIBBONS

Page 1

"*This is the net . . .*": Andrzej Szczeklik.

three Fates . . . : Robert Graves, *Greek Myths* (London: Penguin Books, 1955), vol. 1, p. 48.

Page 2

"*a soft, deceiving sash . . .*": Roberto Calasso, *The Marriage of Cadmus and Harmony*, translated by Tim Parks (New York: Alfred A. Knopf, 1993), p. 100.

The story is told by Er . . . : Plato, *The Republic*, bk. 10, 616b–c, edited by G. R. F. Ferrari, translated by Tom Griffith (Cambridge: Cambridge University Press, 2000).

Page 3

"*through honor or death . . .*": Calasso, *The Marriage of Cadmus and Harmony*, p. 283.

"*true to life . . .*": Seamus Heaney, *Crediting Poetry*, Nobel Lecture, 1995 (Lougherew: Gallery Press, 1995), p. 20.

"*a prayer his body makes entirely . . .*": Seamus Heaney, "St Kevin and the Blackbird," in *The Spirit Level* (London: Faber and Faber, 1996), p. 24.

"*vain, winged tassels*": Calasso, *The Marriage of Cadmus and Harmony*, p. 284.

Page 4

"And that happens regardless of spatial distance . . .": Michał Heller, *Kosmologia Kwantowa* [Quantum Cosmology] (Warsaw: Prószyński i S-ka, 2001), p. 11.

the name Ananke . . . : Calasso, *The Marriage of Cadmus and Harmony,* p. 98.

Page 5

"beacon on the seashore . . .": Juliusz Słowacki, *Beniowski,* canto 1, vv. 68–70, in *Dzieła wszystkie* [Complete Works], edited by J. Kleiner (Wrocław: Zakład Narodowy im. Ossolińskich, 1952–1976), vol. 5, p. 56.

Page 7

"Beneath the ordinary picture . . .": Antoni Kępiński, *Schizofrenia* [Schizophrenia] (Cracow: Wydawnictwo Literackie, 2001), p. 210.

Page 8

the illud tempus . . . : Mircea Eliade, *Myths, Dreams and Mysteries* (New York: Harper and Row, 1975), p. 52.

"We simply don't know . . .": Stefan Chwin, "O rzeczach i o sztuce" [On things and art], *Dekada Literacka,* 2001, no. 7/8, p. 16.

CONSTELLATIONS

Page 9

"break spells . . .": Jerzy Stempowski, *Chimera jak zwierzę pociągowe* [The Chimera as a Beast of Burden] (Warsaw: Czytelnik, 2001), vol. 2, p. 14.

Page 10

"archeus" or "inner alchemist": Paracelsus, *Selected Writings,* edited by Jolande Jacobi, Bollingen Series 28 (Princeton: Princeton University Press, 1998), p. 47.

Page 11

Hamlet's conversation with Polonius: William Shakespeare, *Hamlet,* act 3, scene 2.

Page 12

two of the apostles were on their way to Emmaus: Luke 24:13–35.

"who had looked at her . . .": Denise Levertov, "The Servant-Girl at Emmaus," in *The Stream and the Sapphire: Selected Poems on Religious Themes* (New York: New Directions, 1997), p. 43.

Page 14

In 1951 a British doctor . . . : Richard Ascher, "Münchhausen's Syndrome," *Lancet,* 1951, no. 1:339–341.

Page 17

"*Coming events cast their shadows before*": Thomas Campbell in "Lochiel's Warning," *The Concise Oxford Dictionary of Quotations* (Oxford: Oxford University Press, 1983), p. 60.

Page 18

"*Poetry thus arrived . . .*": Calasso, *The Marriage of Cadmus and Harmony*, p. 144.

"*Tell all the truth . . .*": Emily Dickinson, *The Poems of Emily Dickinson* (Cambridge: Harvard University Press, Belknap Press, 1999), p. 494.

"*making pronouncements is difficult . . .*": Władysław Szumowski, *Historia medycyny filozoficznie ujęta* [The History of Medicine Philosophically Expressed], 3rd edition (Cracow: Sanmedia, 1994), p. 80.

Page 20

"*He who does not take control . . .*": Paracelsus, *Selected Writings*, p. 150.

THE ELIXIR OF LIFE

Page 21

The birth of Asclepius: Robert Graves, *Greek Myths*, pp. 173–175.

Page 23

"*heavenly alchemy*": William Shakespeare, sonnet 33.

"*posed as a sacred science . . .*": Mircea Eliade, *The Forge and the Crucible*, translated by Stephen Corrin (Chicago: University of Chicago Press, 1962), p. 9.

"*Very early on . . .*": Ibid., p. 8.

Page 24

regressus ad uterum: Jean Chevalier and Alain Gheerbrant, *The Penguin Dictionary of Symbols*, translated by J. Buchanan-Brown (London: Penguin Books, 1996), p. 12.

"*Transform yourselves . . .*": Eliade, *The Forge and the Crucible*, p. 158.

Page 25

John Ripley: Ibid., p. 163.

"*just a Promethean dream . . .*": Czesław Miłosz, "Treatise on Theology," in *Second Space: New Poems*, translated by Czesław Miłosz and Robert Hass (New York: Harper Collins, Ecco Press, 2004), p. 57.

Page 26

"*inextinguishable laughter*": Calasso, *The Marriage of Cadmus and Harmony*, p. 95.

Page 29

"second childishness . . .": William Shakespeare, *As You Like It,* act 2, scene 7.

Page 30

If aging cells. . . : Constance Holden, "The Quest to Reverse Time's Toll," *Science* 295, no. 5557 (2002): 1032.

A TANGLE OF SERPENTS

Page 33

"amid the silence . . .": Jan Parandowski, *Mitologia* [Mythology], 5th edition (Warsaw: Czytelnik, 1950), p. 146.

Page 35

"The Lord said to Moses . . .": Exodus 4: 1–4.
"He who holds . . .": Stanisław Wyspiański, *Wyzwolenie* [Deliverance], act 3, vv. 601–602, in *Dramaty* [Tragedies] (Cracow: Wydawnictwo Literackie, 1955), p. 502.

Page 37

"The children would play . . .": Władysław Kopaliński, *Słownik symboli* [A Dictionary of Symbols] (Warsaw: Wiedza Powszechna, 1990), p. 448.
"I will put enmity . . .": Genesis 3: 15.
"But never met this Fellow . . .": Dickinson, *The Poems of Emily Dickinson,* p. 443.

Page 40

"that was furthest . . .": Calasso, *The Marriage of Cadmus and Harmony,* pp. 199–200.

IN BETWEEN ART AND SCIENCE

Page 42

"a confession of the body": Oscar V. de L. Milosz, "Canticle of Knowledge" in *The Noble Traveller,* edited by Christopher Bamford (West Stockbridge, Mass.: Lindisfarne Books, 1985), p. 181.
"the color, shape, size . . .": Szumowski, *Historia medycyny filozoficznie ujęta,* p. 101.
"a dissection every day . . .": Vivian Nutton, "Logic, Learning and Experimental Medicine," *Science* 295, no. 5556 (2002): 800–801.

Page 43

"I shall not keep . . .": Meyer Friedman and Gerald W. Friedland, *Medicine's 10 Greatest Discoveries* (New Haven: Yale University Press, 1998), p. 4.

"that corpse would never rise from the dead": Fyodor Dostoyevsky, *The Idiot*, translated by Constance Garnett (Norwalk, Conn.: Heritage Press, 1956), pp. 366–367.

Page 44

"death has lent shockingly large dimensions": Maria Rzepińska, *Siedem wieków malarstwa europejskiego* [Seven Centuries of European Painting] (Wrocław: Zakład Narodowy im. Ossolińskich, 1988), p. 262.

Page 45

"silently grouped around the marble slab table": Stefan Chwin, *Death in Danzig*, translated by Philip Boehm (Orlando, Fla.: Harcourt Books, 2004), p. 10.

Pages 45–46

"All science is either physics or stamp collecting": Andrzej Białas, "Nauka i medycyna" [Science and medicine], *Medycyna Praktyczna*, 1999, no. 6:15–17.

Page 46

"identification" principle: Andrzej Staruszkiewicz, "O najważniejszej z nauk" [On the most important of the sciences], in *Rozmowy na nowy wiek 1* [Conversations for the New Century 1], by Katarzyna Janowska and Piotr Mucharski (Cracow: Wydawnictwo Znak, 2001), pp. 251–265.

Page 47

"They are unchanging . . .": Władysław Tatarkiewicz, *Historia filozofii* [A History of Philosophy], 17th edition (Warsaw: PWN, 1999), vol. 1, p. 48.

Paul Dirac once said . . .: Marc Lachieze-Rey and Jean-Pierre Luminet, *Celestial Treasury: From the Music of the Spheres to the Conquest of Space*, translated by Joe Laredo (Cambridge: Cambridge University Press, 2001), p. 57.

"provide only abstract images . . .": Ibid., p. 2.

Page 48

origins problem: John L. Casti, "The World of Testable Truths," *Nature* 414, no. 6861 (2001): 254.

Page 49

Further reading on prostacyclin: (a) The discovery of prostacyclin: R. J. Gryglewski, S. Bunting, S. Moncada, R. J. Flower, and J. R. Vane, "Arterial Walls Are Protected against Deposition of Platelet Thrombi by a Substance (Prostaglandin X) Which They Make from Prostaglandin Endoperoxide," *Prostaglandins* 12 (1976): 685–713. (b) Actions of prostacyclin in man: A. Szczeklik, R. J. Gryglewski, E. Niżankowska, R. Niżankowski, J. Musiał, R. Piętoń, and J. Mruk, "Circulatory and Anti-platelet Effects of Intravenous Prostacyclin in Healthy

Man," *Pharmacological Research Communications* 10 (1978): 545–566. (c) First therapeutic application: A. Szczeklik, R. Niżankowski, S. Skawiński, J. Szczeklik, P. Głuszko, and R. Gryglewski, "Successful Therapy of Advanced Arteriosclerosis Obliterans with Prostacyclin," *Lancet* 1 (1979): 1111–1115.

Page 50

our colleagues at the hospital: The doctors from our hospital who received the first shots of prostacyclin were Jacek Musiał, Rafał Niżankowski, Ryszard Piętoń, and Józef Mruk.

Page 51

"selfish genes": Richard Dawkins, *The Selfish Gene* (Oxford: Oxford University Press, 1976).

"the individual organism . . .": Richard Dawkins, *Unweaving the Rainbow* (London: Penguin Books, 1998), pp. 308–309.

Page 52

"systems that cannot easily be brought closer . . .": Białas, "Nauka i medycyna."

"The whole, considered in relation to its parts . . .": Józef Życiński, *Bóg i ewolucja* [God and Evolution] (Lublin: TN KUL, 2002), p. 114.

"The whole is more than the sum of the parts": Cited in John L. Casti, *Complexification* (London: Abacus, 1994), p. 171.

Page 53

"It is not for art . . .": Zbigniew Herbert, "The Ornament Makers," translated by John and Bogdana Carpenter, *Salmagundi,* Winter–Spring 1999, no. 121–122:74.

According to Henryk Elzenberg . . . : Henryk Elzenberg, "Nauka i barbarzyństwo" [Science and barbarism] in *Z historii filozofii* [From the History of Philosophy] (Cracow: Wydawnictwo Znak, 1995), pp. 218–230.

"to give . . . certain, clear knowledge . . .": Zbigniew Herbert, *Still Life with a Bridle,* translated by John and Bogdana Carpenter (Hopewell, N.J.: Ecco Press, 1991), p. 150.

a sculpture dedicated to his memory: It is by Karol Gąsienica-Szostak.

Piwnica pod Baranami: The cabaret is named after its location on Cracow's marketplace, in the "Wine cellar at the sign of the rams."—Translator

Page 54

"The truth is a mobile army of metaphors": Friedrich Nietzsche, *Über Wahrheit und Lüge im aussermoralischen Sinne* [On Truth and Lies in an Extramoral Sense], in *Werke,* vol. 3, pt. 2 (1972), cited in Roberto Calasso, *Literature and Gods* (New York: A. Knopf, 2001), p. 184.

THE RHYTHM OF THE HEART

Page 60

"*with a subtle rhythmic anxiety*": Ł. Kamieński (1918), quoted in Mieczysław Tomaszewski, *Chopin* (Poznań: Wydawnictwo Podsiedlik-Reniowski i S-ka, 1998), p. 284.

"*when its crown bends . . .*": Franz Liszt, quoted in Tomaszewski, *Chopin*, p. 288.

Page 61

discreet deviations . . . : J. and M. Sobieski (1960), quoted in Tomaszewski, *Chopin*, p. 284.

Dorland's Medical Dictionary, 29th edition (Philadelphia: Saunders Company, 2000).

Page 67

The Oxford Companion to Music, by Percy Alfred Scholes, 10th edition (Oxford: Oxford University Press, 1984), p. 872.

"*binds together distant shores . . .*": Zbigniew Herbert, "Attempt at a Description," translated by Czesław Miłosz, in *Selected Poems* (London: Penguin Books, 1968), p. 103.

A PURIFYING POWER

Page 68

vis medicatrix naturae: W. F. Bynum, "Nature's Helping Hand," *Nature* 414, no. 6859 (2001): 21.

Page 69

"*in contemporary language . . .*": Władysław Tatarkiewicz, *Historia estetyki* [A History of Aesthetics] (Wrocław: Zakład Narodowy im. Ossolińskich, 1960), p. 30.

Pseudo-Plutarch, *De Musica*, cited in Tatarkiewicz, *Historia estetyki*, p. 24.

Page 70

The Pythagoreans believed . . . : Enrico Fubini, *The History of Music Aesthetics*, translated by Michael Hatwell (London: Macmillan, 1991), p. 25.

"*The Pythagoreans . . . cleansed the body by means of medicine*": Władysław Tatarkiewicz, *Estetyka starożytna* [Ancient Aesthetics] (Wrocław: Zakład Narodowy im. Ossolińskich, 1960), p. 94.

"*amputated by an unknown censor*": Alexandre Nicev, *L'enigme de la catharsis tragique dans Aristotle* (Sofia: Bulgarian Academy of Sciences, 1970), p. 6.

Page 71

"one of the most difficult concepts . . .": Chevalier and Gheerbrant, *The Penguin Dictionary of Symbols*, p. 563.

"boundless awe": Roberto Calasso, *Ka,* translated by Tim Parks (New York: A. A. Knopf, 1998), pp. 149–150.

"It is impossible for any number . . .": Keith Devlin, *Mathematics: The Science of Patterns* (New York: Scientific American Library, 1997), p. 29.

Page 72

"Fermat's last theorem was a theorem at last": Ibid., p. 208.

"it is doubtful if . . .": Ibid., p. 200.

"the equation $z^n = x^n + y^n$ . . .": Ibid., pp. 29–30. (The power n is not only greater than 2, but an integer as well. Mathematicians ignore the trivial solutions that arise when one of the unknowns is allowed to be zero.)

"Tragedy is an imitation of an action . . .": Aristotle, *The Poetics*, translated by S. H. Butcher, 4th edition (London: Macmillan, 1923), bk. 6, 2.

"In other words, the sublimation . . .": Tatarkiewicz, *Estetyka starożytna*, p. 147.

Page 73

iatreia kai katharsis: Aristotle, *Politics* 7, 1341b, 32–1342a, 11–15.

"a natural psychological and biological process": Tatarkiewicz, *Historia estetyki*, p. 147.

"Sounds find a resonance . . .": Tatarkiewicz, *Estetyka starożytna*, p. 91.

"upon their disorganised souls . . .": Eric Weiner and Isaiah Sonne, *The Philosophy and Theory of Music in Judaeo-Arabic Literature*, cited in Curt Sachs, *The Rise of Music in the Ancient World* (New York: Norton, 1943), p. 253.

Page 74

the choir of old men in Euripides: *The Oxford Companion to Classical Civilisation*, edited by Simon Hornblower and Antony Spawforth (Oxford: Oxford University Press, 1998), p. 477.

"Protect us from an empty life . . .": Józef Czechowicz, "Modlitwa żałobna" [Requiem prayer], in *Wybór wierszy* [Selected Poems] (Lublin: Wydawnictwo Lubelskie, 1974), p. 184.

"in a matter as morally and socially important as music . . .": Władysław Tatarkiewicz, *Dzieje sześciu pojęć* [The History of Six Concepts] (Warsaw: PWN, 1976), pp. 210–212.

Page 75

"a moderate and settled temper": Aristotle, *Metaphysics,* quoted in Sachs, *The Rise of Music in the Ancient World,* p. 248.

"What made Dorian . . .": Sachs, *The Rise of Music in the Ancient World,* p. 248.

"the Mixolydian and hyper-Lydian modes . . .": Cited in Jamie James, *The Music of the Spheres* (London: Abacus, 1995), p. 57.

Page 76

"was suffering from the bane of insomnia . . .": Julia Hartwig, "Drogi Goldberg" [Dear Goldberg] in *Zawsze od nowa* [Over and Over Again] (Warsaw: Wydawnictwo Twój Styl, 1999), p. 62.
"a golden vessel . . .": Ibid.

Page 77

"the built-in preordained universal": Cited in Mark Jude Tramo, "Music of the Hemispheres," *Science* 291, no. 5501 (2001): 54–56.
"many different types of scales . . .": Patricia M. Gray et al., "The Music of Nature and the Nature of Music," *Science* 291, no. 5501 (2001): 52.

Page 78

"Every disease is a musical problem . . .": Cited in Oliver Sacks, *A Leg to Stand On* (New York: Summit Books, 1984), p. 137.

SUFFERING

Page 80

"poses to the human mind . . .": John Paul II, *Ewangelia cierpienia* [The Gospel of Suffering] (Cracow: Wydawnictwo Znak, 1997), p. 167.
"Who committed the sin . . .": John 9: 1–3.
"exorcism of pain from the world": Stefan Chwin, "O bólu" [On pain], in *Rozmowy na koniec wieku 3* [Conversations for the End of the Century 3], by Katarzyna Janowska and Piotr Mucharski (Cracow: Wydawnictwo Znak, 1999), p. 83.

Page 81

"willow delights in . . .": J. R. Vane, R. M. Botting, editors, *Aspirin and Other Salicylates* (London: Chapman and Hall, 1992), pp. 3–4.

Page 82

"Non interesse quod . . .": Szumowski, *Historia medycyny filozoficznie ujęta*, p. 98.
revelers: A. S. Lyons and R. J. Petrucelli, *Medicine: An Illustrated History* (New York: Abradale Press and Harry N. Abrams, 1987), p. 528.
"A fluid that pervades the entire universe . . .": Ibid., p. 484.

Page 83

"fixed it with bonds that could not be untied . . .": Calasso, *The Marriage of Cadmus and Harmony*, p. 147.

Page 84

"break so vast a Heart": Dickinson, poem 1308, in *The Poems of Emily Dickinson*, p. 506.

"After great pain . . .": Dickinson, poem 372, in *The Poems of Emily Dickinson*, p. 170.

Page 85

"spiritual medicine": John Paul II, *Ewangelia cierpienia*, p. 92.

"To comfort someone means . . .": Henryk Elzenberg, *Kłopot z istnieniem* [The Trouble with Existence] (Cracow: Wydawnictwo Znak, 1994), p. 82.

"Humanity undergoes a Calvary of suffering": John Paul II, *Ewangelia cierpienia*, p. 57.

"Could God have justified Himself . . .": John Paul II, *Crossing the Threshold of Hope* (New York: A. A. Knopf, 1994), chap. 10.

Page 86

the "Heavenly Doctor": John Paul II, *Ewangelia cierpienia*, p. 67.

Page 87

"Cure her of that . . .": William Shakespeare, *Macbeth*, act 5, scene 3.

Page 88

"reality with a thousand faces . . .": John Paul II, *Ewangelia cierpienia*, p. 73.

EXITUS

Page 90

"Like a string when the concert's over": Zbigniew Herbert, "Ostatnie słowa" [Last words], *Zeszyty Literackie* 72 (2001): 5.

"I've seen a Dying Eye . . .": Dickinson, poem 648, in *The Poems of Emily Dickinson*, p. 290.

Page 91

"Is it only then . . .": Henryka Łazowertówna, "Imiona światła" [The names of light], in *Od Kochanowskiego do Staffa: Antologia lyriki polskiej* [An Anthology of Polish Poetry from Kochanowski to Staff], edited by Wacław Borowy (Warsaw: PIW, 1958), p. 382.

Page 92

"The supreme diplomat of the century": J. W. von Goethe, *Collections des portraits historiques de M. le Baron Gérard*, in *Werke* (Zürich: Artemis, 1954), vol. 13, p. 993.

"would have got under his skin . . .": François René de Chateaubriand, *Mémoires d'outre-tombe* (Paris: Gallimard, 1958), vol. 2, p. 901.

"Our dear friend, the eternal traitor Talleyrand . . .": The Duchess d'Abrantès, "Salon de Monsieur de Talleyrand," in "Histoire de salons de Paris," *L'advocat* (Paris) 6 (1838): 1.

"There's nothing I fear so much as improper protocol": Charles Augustin Saint-Beuve, "Talleyrand," in *Nouveaux lundis* (Paris: Calman Lévy, 1844), vol. 12, p. 112.

Page 93

"in the bosom of the Roman Catholic Apostolic Church": Roberto Calasso, *The Ruin of Kasch* (London: Vintage, 1995), p. 347.

"Every wish will diminish me . . .": Honoré de Balzac, *The Wild Ass's Skin*, translated by Herbert J. Hunt (London: Penguin Books, 1995), p. 51.

Page 94

"to preempt the final blow": Chwin, "O bólu," p. 77.

"doubly at home": Bishop J. Pietraszko, *Nasze powroty do Chrystusa* [Our Returns to Christ] (Cracow: Wydawnictwo św. Stanisława Archidiecezji Krakowskiej, 2001), p. 50.

"the final climb up the rocky chimneystack": Ibid., p. 151.

Pages 94–95

"All the great Parisian ladies . . .": Pauline Viardot-Garcia, quoted in Jarosław Iwaszkiewicz, *Chopin* (Cracow: PWM, 1995), p. 349.

Page 95

"The artist's sister . . .": Cyprian K. Norwid, quoted in Iwaszkiewicz, *Chopin*, p. 342.

In his final hours Chopin . . . : There are a large number of medical essays on Chopin's illness. Recent examples include J. C. Davila, "Étude de la maladie de Chopin à travers sa correspondence" (thèse pour le doctorat en médecine, University of Toulouse III, 1995).

"still found the strength . . .": Viardot-Garcia, quoted in Tomaszewski, *Chopin*, p. 124.

"Do it for me . . .": Ibid.

"from the land of Mozart . . .": Heinrich Heine, quoted in Tomaszewski, *Chopin*, p. 77.

Page 97

In a long list from ten Dutch hospitals . . . : Pim van Lommel et al., "Near-Death Experience in Survivors of Cardiac Arrest: A Prospective Study in the Netherlands," *Lancet* 358, no. 9298 (2001): 2039–2045.

Page 98

"the transformation of the living into specters . . .": Maria Janion, *Żyjąc tracimy życie* [We Lose Life by Living] (Warsaw: Wydawnictwo W.A.B., 2001), p. 48.

"how before our very eyes . . .": Ibid., p. 40.

"in a prison with windows but no doors": Oliver Sacks, *Awakenings* (New York: Vintage Books, 1999).

"I, Her the Armenian . . .": Juliusz Słowacki, *Król-Duch* [King-Spirit], canto 1, v. 10, in *Dzieła wszystkie,* p. 146.

"on the tenth day . . .": Plato, *The Republic,* bk. 10, 614b.

Page 99

"bold step": David K. C. Cooper and Denton A. Cooley, "Christian Neethling Barnard, 1922–2001," *Circulation* 104, no. 7327 (2001): 2756–2757.

Page 100

Although he could feel the cardiac surgeons breathing down his neck . . .: Raymond Hoffenberg, "Christian Barnard: His First Transplants and Their Impact on Concepts of Death," *BMJ* 323, no. 7327 (2001): 1478–1480.

Page 101

"God speaks to each of us . . .": Rainer Maria Rilke, *Das Buch vom mönchischen Leben* [The Book of Monastic Life] in *Das Stundenbuch* [The Book of Hours] (1899).

"In the course of this fugue . . .": Douglas Hofstadter, *Gödel, Escher, Bach: An Eternal Golden Braid* (London: Vintage Books, 1980), p. 80.

CHIMERA

Page 103

"From then on . . .": Edward S. Golub and Douglas R. Green, *Immunology: A Synthesis* (Sunderland, Mass.: Sinauer Associates, 1991), p. 6.

Page 104

"Today I am going to tell you a thing . . .": Ibid., p. 3.

Page 105

"I can't catch human smallpox . . .": Szumowski, *Historia medycyny filozoficznie ujęta,* p. 532.

Page 106

"from top to bottom . . .": Ibid., p. 274.

Page 107

"the plague bacillus never dies . . .": Albert Camus, *The Plague,* translated by Stuart Gilbert (New York: Alfred A. Knopf, 1968), p. 278.

"Of the three most eminent doctors . . .": Tomaszewski, *Chopin,* p. 81.

"We have to rest . . .": Thomas Mann, *The Magic Mountain*, translated by John E. Woods (New York: Alfred. A. Knopf, 1995), p. 71.

Page 108

"A scrap of life . . .": Jerzy Liebert, "Kołysanka jodłowa" [Fir-tree lullaby] in Borowy, *Od Kochanowskiego do Staffa*, p. 374.

"other factors, principally natural selection . . .": R. P. O. Davies et al., "Historical Declines in Tuberculosis in England and Wales: Improving Social Conditions or Natural Selection?" *International Journal of Tuberculosis and Lung Disease* 3, no. 12 (1999): 1051–1054.

Page 109

"the gas-ridden, overcrowded trenches . . .": John Oxford, "Nature's Biological Weapon," *Nature* 429, no. 6990 (2004): 345–346.

Page 110

"but in raw numbers influenza killed . . .": J. M. Barry, *The Great Influenza: The Epic Story of the Deadliest Plague in History* (New York: Viking, 2004), p. 4.

Page 111

Homer described the Chimera . . . : *The Iliad of Homer*, translated by Richmond Lattimore (Chicago: University of Chicago Press, 1961), bk. 6, line 181.

"a bastard of the imagination": Zbigniew Herbert, "Pegaz" [Pegasus], in *Król mrówek* [The King of the Ants] (Cracow: Wydawnictwo a5, 2001), p. 108.

Page 113

the Chimera implies the epithet "beast of burden": Stempowski, *Chimera jak zwierzę pociągowe*.

AFTER THE GENOME

Page 116

"without wanting to be held back by the boundaries of an identity": Calasso, *The Marriage of Cadmus and Harmony*, p. 174.

Page 117

"susceptibility genes": Trisha Gura, "Can SNPs Deliver on Susceptibility Genes?" *Science* 293, no. 5530 (2001): 593–595.

"Thus, from a genomic perspective . . .": Svante Pääbo, "The Mosaic That Is Our Genome," *Nature* 421, no. 6921 (2003): 409–412.

Page 119

"Such was Proteus . . .": Jan Kochanowski, "Do gór i lasów" [To the mountains and forests], in Borowy, *Od Kochanowskiego do Staffa,* p. 2.

Page 120

"Omnis cellula e cellula": Rudolf Virchow, quoted in Anne McLaren, "Cloning: Pathways to a Pluripotent Future," *Science* 288, no. 5472 (2000): 1775–1780.

"thought experiment": Hans Spemann, *Embryonic Development and Induction* (New Haven, Conn.: Yale University Press, 1938).

"What is now proved . . .": William Blake, *The Marriage of Heaven and Hell,* plate 8, in *The Poetry and Prose of William Blake,* edited by David V. Erdman (Garden City, N.Y.: Doubleday and Company, 1968), p. 36.

Page 121

"later twin": Dan W. Brock, "Human Cloning and Our Sense of Self," *Science* 296, no. 5566 (2002): 314–316.

Page 122

"becoming a mermaid, half-woman and half-fish": P. Anversa, M. Sussman, and R. Bolli, "Molecular Genetic Advances in Cardiovascular Medicine: Focus on the Myocyte," *Circulation* 109 (2004): 2832–2838.

"Stem-cell therapy provides . . .": A. Mathur, J. F. Martin, "Stem Cell and Repair of the Heart," *Lancet* 364 (2004): 183–192.

Page 123

"No Saturdays . . .": Woo Suk Hwang et al., "Evidence of Pluripotent Human Embryonic Stem Cell Line Derived from a Cloned Blastocyst," *Science* 303, no. 5664 (2004): 1669–1674.

Page 124

For more on the Korean experiments on stem cells, see also David Cyranoski, "Stem-Cell Research: Crunch Time for Korea's Cloners," *Nature* 429, no. 6987 (2004): 12–14.

Page 125

"post-human world": Francis Fukuyama, *Our Post-human Future: Consequences of the Biotechnology Revolution* (New York: Farrar, Strauss and Giroux, 2002).

Page 126

"decayed relics . . .": T. A. Brown, *Genomes* (BIOS Scientific Publishers, 1999), p. 138.

"The barren desert . . .": John C. Avise, "Evolving Genomic Metaphors: A New Look at the Language of DNA," *Science* 294, no. 5540 (2001): 86–87.

Page 127

"the archaeological excavation . . .": Marek Sanak, *Podstawy medycyny molekularnej* [Foundations of Molecular Medicine] (Cracow: Medycyna Praktyczna, 2001), p. 93.

"should be called not junk DNA . . .": Wojciech Makalowski, "Not Junk after All," *Science* 300, no. 5623 (2003): 1246–1247.

"evolutionary through and through": Michał Heller, *Sens życia i sens wszechświata* [The Meaning of Life and the Meaning of the Universe] (Tarnów: Biblos, 2002), p. 137.

Page 128

"The scientific theory of evolution . . .": Ibid.
"a considerable number of theologians and clergy": Ibid., p. 135.
"man does not want to accept the truth . . .": Życiński, *Bóg i ewolucja*, p. 165.
"epistemological abuses": Ibid., p. 44.
"The battles among genes . . .": Czesław Miłosz, "Scientists," in Miłosz, *Second Space: New Poems*, p. 25.
"selfish gene": Dawkins, *The Selfish Gene*.

Page 129

"the disclaimers are brief . . .": Mary Midgley, *Science and Poetry* (London: Routledge, 2001), p. 195.
"Organisms and their environment evolve . . .": James Lovelock, "Gaia: The Living Earth," *Nature* 426, no. 6968 (2003): 769–770.
"makes man His confidant . . .": Życiński, *Bóg i ewolucja*, p. 197.

Page 130

"cooperation and symbiosis that drive evolution": Lynn Margulis and Dorian Sagan, *Acquiring Genomes: A Theory of the Origin of the Species* (New York: Basic Books, 2002), p. 156.
"linear time extending infinitely backwards and forwards": Czesław Miłosz, introduction to O. V. de L. Milosz, *The Noble Traveller*, p. 40.

ALTERATIONS AND RETURNS

Page 133

"As the fog of human-resources jargon . . .": Richard Horton, "The Doctor's Role in Advocacy," *Lancet* 359, no. 9305 (2002): 458.
Physician's Charter: Medycyna Praktyczna, 2002, special edition 4; see also

"Medical Professionalism in the New Millennium: A Physician's Charter,"
Lancet 359, no. 9305 (2002): 520–522.

Page 135

"the doctor always washes his hands . . .": Hugo Steinhaus, *Słownik racjonalny*
[A Rational Dictionary] (Wrocław: Zakład Narodowy im. Ossolińskich, 1992),
p. 73.

When Alexander the Great . . .: Quintus Curtius Rufus, *The History of Alexander*, translated by John Yardley (London: Penguin Books, 1984), pp. 34–35.

Page 136

"The ability to reproduce . . .": Daniel E. Koshland Jr, "The Seven Pillars of
Life," *Science* 295, no. 5563 (2002): 2215–2216.

Erwin Schrödinger, *What Is Life?* Cambridge University Press, Cambridge
1944.

"neither original, nor up-to-date, nor accurate . . .": Richard Rorty, "Studied
Ambiguity," *Science* 293, no. 5539 (2001): 2399–2400.

Page 137

"Living matter . . .": Quoted in Brian Ridley, *On Science* (London: Routledge,
2001), p. 50.

"studied ambiguity": Rorty, "Studied Ambiguity."

"a capricious line of repetitions . . .": Vladimir Nabokov, quoted in Mariusz
Wilk, "Dziennik północny" [Northern diary], *Rzeczpospolita*, 13–14 April 2002,
p. A8.

Page 138

"nature is rich . . .": Ridley, *On Science*, p. 34.

"asking about reality at its deepest level": Roger Penrose, *The Road to Reality: A
Complete Guide to the Laws of the Universe* (London: Jonathan Cape, 2004),
p. 1028.

"only in the inner life . . .": Adam Zagajewski, "Against Poetry," address delivered at the meeting I Dialoghi di San Giorgio, 15–17 September 2004, Giorgio
Cini Foundation, Venice.

Page 141

Francis Crick . . .: György Buzsáki, "Interconnected Stories of Brain Rhythms,"
Science 294, no. 5550 (2001): 2295–2297.

"the person within": Antonio Damasio, "Mental Self: The Person Within,"
Nature 423, no. 6973 (2003): 227.

"you must give yourself . . .": John Paul II, *Ewangelia cierpienia*, p. 318.

Page 142

"I am different . . .": Paracelsus, *Selected Writings*, p. 3.

"art is the conjuration . . .": Julia Hartwig, "Jest i tym" [It's this too] in *Zawsze od nowa,* p. 121.

Page 143

"you see the world . . .": Adam Zagajewski, "The Greenhouse," in *Mysticism for Beginners,* translated by Clare Cavanagh (New York: Farrar Straus and Giroux, 1997).

"instead of many roles . . .": Kępiński, *Schizofrenia,* p. 178.